WHOLE WOMAN

HOMEOPATHY

THE COMPREHENSIVE GUIDE TO TREATING PMS, MENOPAUSE, CYSTITIS, AND OTHER PROBLEMS— NATURALLY AND EFFECTIVELY

JUDYTH REICHENBERG-ULLMAN, N.D., M.S.W.

PRIMA HEALTH
A Division of Prima Publishing
3000 LAVA RIDGE COURT • ROSEVILLE, CALIFORNIA 95661
(800) 632-8676 • www.primahealth.com

Warning—Disclaimer
This book is not intended to provide medical advice and is sold with the understanding that the publisher and the author are not liable for the misconception or misuse of information provided. The author and Prima Publishing shall have neither liability nor responsibility to any person or entity with respect to any loss, damage, or injury caused or alleged to be caused directly or indirectly by the information contained in this book or the use of any products mentioned. Readers should not use any of the products discussed in this book without the advice of a medical professional.

PRIMA PUBLISHING, the PRIMA COLOPHON, and PRIMA HEALTH are registered trademarks of Prima Communications Inc., registered in the United States and other countries.

Pseudonyms have been used throughout to protect the privacy of the individuals involved.
All products mentioned in this book are trademarks of their respective companies.

Library of Congress Cataloging-in-Publication Data
Reichenberg-Ullman, Judyth.
    Whole woman homeopathy : the comprehensive guide to treating PMS, menopause, cystitis, and other problems—naturally and effectively / Judyth Reichenberg-Ullman.
       p. cm.
    Includes bibliographical references and index.
    ISBN 0-7615-2411-8
1. Generative organs, Female—Diseases—Homeopathic treatment. 2. Women—Diseases—Homeopathic treatment. I. Title.

RX465.R45 2000   CIP
618.1'06—dc21   00-035648

00 01 02 03 DD 10 9 8 7 6 5 4 3 2 1

Printed in the United States of America

HOW TO ORDER
Single copies may be ordered from Prima Publishing, 3000 Lava Ridge Court, Roseville, CA 95661; telephone (800) 632-8676 ext. 4444. Quantity discounts are also available. On your letterhead, include information concerning the intended use of the books and the number of books you wish to purchase.

Visit us online at www.primahealth.com

To women everywhere who embody courage, wisdom, beauty, strength, compassion, and depth of spirit. May this book offer you inspiration and hope in your journey to total and ultimate healing.

Contents

Foreword by Dr. Susan Lark   vii

Acknowledgments   ix

Introduction: Sharing My Story   x

PART ONE
Homeopathy and Women: A Perfect Match

1. Healing the Whole Woman: You Are Far More Than the Sum of Your Body Parts   3
2. Drugs, Surgery, or Hormones—What Is Your Pleasure?: What Conventional Medicine Has to Offer You   9
3. Homeopathy—What It Is and How It Can Help You: A Safe and Effective Natural Approach   17
4. Why Many Women Choose Homeopathy over Conventional Medicine: Compelling Reasons to Make Homeopathy Your Medicine of Choice   28
5. How Homeopathy and Conventional Medicine Can Work Hand in Hand: A Compatible Relationship If Both Partners Are Willing   36
6. When to Treat Yourself and When You Need a Homeopath   43

PART TWO
Healing Yourself with Homeopathy
for Acute Women's Problems

7. Taking an Acute Homeopathic Case: Knowing How to Ask the Right Questions   51

8. Choosing the Best Homeopathic Medicine: The Closer the Match, the Better the Result   58
9. Once You Have Selected a Medicine: How, When, and How Often to Take It   61
10. Your Women's Homeopathic Self-Care Medicine Kit: Make Sure You Have the Medicines You Need   67
11. Conditions You Can Self-Treat Safely and Effectively   70

PART THREE
Homeopathic Care from a Professional

12. What Every Woman Needs to Know About Homeopathic Treatment: What to Expect and What Will Be Expected of You   171
13. Conditions for Which You Need a Homeopath   181

PART FOUR
Materia Medica

14. Fifty Homeopathic Medicines for Women's Acute Self-Care   275

PART FIVE
Enhancing Your Healing

15. Complements to Homeopathic Healing: Essential Elements of a Balanced Lifestyle   331
16. The Promise of Healing the Whole You: What If You Were Completely Healed?   336

Appendix: Expanding Your Knowledge of Homeopathy   339

Notes   343

Glossary   345

Index   347

About the Author   355

Foreword

Now more than ever, women are taking an active role in their health care. A generation ago, changing doctors, finding a female physician, or getting a second opinion were almost unheard of. In sharp contrast, women today are not afraid to question their doctors' recommendations and do not hesitate to refuse what they consider to be potentially harmful drugs, surgeries, and interventions. And now the search for a quick fix is being replaced by a desire for a deeply effective, long-lasting, holistic approach to healing. With a heightened awareness of the body-mind-spirit connection, women are no longer satisfied with being treated merely as bodies, but insisting that their entire being be honored, addressed, and healed.

As a result, over the past two decades the demand for natural medicine has flourished. Various studies estimate that up to a third of the population of the United States uses some form of alternative therapy. And it is no wonder that natural medicine is so popular, especially with women who are seeking safer, more natural treatment options. Side effects are minimal compared with conventional medications. Once women learn that there are often effective, nontoxic alternatives to drugs and surgery, such as herbs, diet, homeopathy, and yoga, they open a door to a world of unlimited healing opportunities. In addition to being safe, natural medicines can be highly effective.

There are many women's conditions for which conventional medicine does not have an effective, universally acceptable, or permanent solution. Take endometriosis for example. Conventional research has not yet definitively found the cause of this problem, but the results of the orthodox treatments may be worse than the original symptoms. Standard interventions typically include one or more surgeries and suppression of ovulation by drugs that can only be used for short periods of time due to their severe side effects. Women who take these medications are thrown into a temporary state of menopause complete with hot flashes and loss of bone density. Conventional medicine offers no sure cure for PMS, miscarriages, infertility, and for breast, uterine, and, particularly, ovarian cancer. Even simple conditions like bladder infections are treated with antibiotics rather than addressing the underlying cause in order to prevent recurrences.

This is where homeopathic medicine comes in. It is a form of healing that genuinely addresses each woman as an integrated whole. Safe and gentle, homeopathy is so effective in many cases that one dose can last for months at a time. And homeopathy is a user-friendly type of medicine—a wide number of acute conditions, including bladder infections, vaginal infections, and morning sickness, can respond beautifully and rapidly to self-treatment. More chronic conditions, such as PMS, hot flashes, and menstrual problems of all kinds, can be helped, sometimes dramatically, under the care of an experienced homeopathic physician or practitioner.

Whole Woman Homeopathy offers a wealth of practical information drawn from the author's sixteen years of practice as a naturopathic and homeopathic physician and her prior experience as a psychiatric social worker. Judyth Reichenberg-Ullman is one of the most well-known homeopaths in this country, treating patients from all over the United States and abroad. As a clinician, teacher, and author, she aspires to make homeopathy understandable and accessible for patients and physicians alike. You will find this book an invaluable addition to your women's health-care library. Not only does Dr. Reichenberg-Ullman provide explicit instructions on self-care for many common women's problems, but she also shares her patients' stories, in their own words, of how homeopathy has changed their lives. In addition to the comprehensive information on homeopathy, she includes specific naturopathic recommendations for diet, nutritional supplements, herbs, and lifestyle for each of the forty-five conditions covered in this book.

Whole Woman Homeopathy is the most comprehensive and practical book that I have seen on homeopathic care for women. I hope that many women read it, use it as a reference, share it with family and friends, and find it to be of inspiration in their own healing journeys.

Susan M. Lark, M.D.

Acknowledgments

I thank all of those in my life who have taught me so much about what it means to be a woman. My supportive, wise, and extraordinarily patient and good-humored husband, Bob, for encouraging me in my healing work for myself and my patients and, above all, for loving me for better or for worse. My dear mother, Essie, who is no longer with us, for her never-ending love and for always telling me how thrilled she was to see me. My dearest friends, especially Wahaba, Sheila, and Randa, for being there when I need them. The women I have treated as patients over the last sixteen years, who have taught me, and continue to teach me, so much every day. The teachers, students, colleagues, and healers who have inspired me in countless ways. The courageous women who, like myself, have faced and overcome the challenge of breast cancer. Many thanks to Dr. Susan Lark, for her willingness to take time out of an already overflowing schedule to write the foreword. I thank my editors at Prima, Susan Silva and Marjorie Lery, for their enthusiasm and support. I am very grateful to Shantimayi for reminding me of what is truly important and lasting in life. And, last but not least, to Jasmine and Truffle, the Golden Retrievers who have curled up by my side and provided unconditional love and amusement as I've birthed this book.

Introduction

SHARING MY STORY

I've wanted to write this book for a long time. The idea first arose in the late '80s and early '90s, when I offered a course called "Healing Women Naturally" in Seattle. The class allowed me to meet many women who yearned for information on how they could address their health issues in a safe, yet effective, way. I was happy that I, as a licensed naturopath physician specializing in homeopathy, could share any wisdom that I had accumulated. As inevitably occurs in any teaching setting, I am sure that I learned as much from my students as they did from me.

The greatest blessing that I have to share with other women is the gift of homeopathy. I once heard that conventional physicians often become disillusioned with their practices because of the lackluster results of their treatments. The experience of being a homeopath is exactly the opposite. Every day I see the profound changes that this remarkable method of healing has brought to my patients' lives. That a form of healing that is so simple and elegant and makes so much common sense to patients can transform lives so powerfully, with doses of a natural medicine administered months or even years apart, still boggles my mind almost as much as it does the minds of my patients.

As far as my own health, I had no gynecological problems at all, not even a single vaginal or bladder infection, until I turned thirty-nine and tried to get pregnant. That led to five miscarriages in five years, despite my cultivating what I considered to be quite a healthful lifestyle. I tried to convince myself that good living, good karma, and sheer willpower could overcome my genetic predisposition (my mother had three miscarriages), but that didn't turn out to be the case. The toll on my body, the excruciating pain of miscarriage number five, and my being nearly forty-five years old caused me and my husband, Bob, to close the chapter on bearing children with a bittersweet mix of regret and relief at moving on to the next phase of our lives.

I was again free of gynecological problems until just before I celebrated my fiftieth birthday, when I was diagnosed with ductal carcinoma in situ (DCIS, a noninvasive, slow-growing form of breast cancer). That experience, which included a mastectomy and free-flap reconstruction, taught me a tremendous amount about love, friends, caring, and what is most important in life.

Although this book is mainly about homeopathy for women, other factors inevitably make their way into the healing relationship. Who we are may be just as healing as whatever medicines we have to offer. A month ago I saw a patient, whom I will call Amanda (also recently diagnosed with DCIS), for her second appointment. We had not yet begun homeopathic treatment. Once Amanda discovered our common diagnosis, during her first appointment, she asked me every question she could about my experience in order to be well-informed about her own choices of treatment. This time, Amanda shared, "You know what was the most helpful of all? To know that it's not my fault. To know that even you, a naturopathic doctor with a natural, healthful lifestyle who had practiced yoga for thirty years, still got breast cancer. That makes me feel so much better. Now I can let go of blaming myself for whatever I might have done wrong to bring this on."

My sincere hope is that this book will introduce women to the beautiful and powerful healing art and science of homeopathy, as well as to our inner healing abilities. Many books exist, with more coming out every day, on the subject of women's health and healing—books that elaborate on the anatomy and physiology of women's gynecological conditions, as well as on conventional and natural (particularly herbal and nutritional) approaches to treatment, and provide psychological and spiritual guidance. Dr. Susan Lark has written many such excellent books and publishes *The Lark Letter,* a monthly newsletter on women's health issues (see appendix). There is no need to duplicate what has already been done extraordinarily well. I share with you, in this book, what I have found to be most effective in healing women during my sixteen years of practice as a homeopath.

My favorite parts of this book are my patients' own stories, which describe how homeopathy has changed their lives in a profound way. For example, Grace, a fifty-seven-year-old Catholic nun from Detroit, shares:

"Thank you for the invitation to contribute to your book. There is so much to say about my experience with you and homeopathy. The best thing that has happened is my new sense of being centered since I began to see you at the age of fifty-four. All of my life, at critical moments, I have been prone to crying, even without any apparent reason. People would tell me I had the gift of tears, but I hated being so vulnerable and never knowing when I would spontaneously start crying. In meetings, classrooms, doctors' offices, family gatherings. Anywhere and everywhere.

Menopause only made matters worse. Crying at the drop of a hat didn't help me gain respect as a professional educator, not to mention the unpredictability of hot flashes and sweats.

"Homeopathy has allowed me to feel so much better, physically, mentally, and emotionally. More energetic, grounded, and at peace with myself. I had no idea that any type of medicine, natural or conventional, could help me feel this stability and harmony. When something interferes with my constitutional homeopathic medicine, I can tell almost immediately, and another dose brings me back into balance. I can honestly say that homeopathy has given me a new life, especially after menopause. Despite the considerable stress of returning to school and entering a new career, I have been remarkably centered and unburdened.

"Besides working with Judyth, I have learned to use a homeopathic home medicine kit to treat myself successfully for ordinary illnesses such as colds and sinus infections. I like them much better than over-the-counter medications and it makes me feel good to know I'm taking something safe and natural. I feel healthy and proud of my life, and I look forward to the years ahead."

Not only does *Whole Woman Homeopathy* contain many other real-life stories of women I have treated with homeopathy (stories that are, wherever possible, told in their own words, though all names have been changed), the book also embraces health conditions that women can self-treat. I have also included a handful of conditions that are not gynecological, per se, but are common to many women. For each condition I have included naturopathic suggestions that I have found consistently effective with my patients over the years. This book's design is intended to be extremely user-friendly to guide you in self-treatment, in selecting a homeopathic medicine, herbs, or other natural treatments that will likely help you quickly and gently.

For some of you reading this book, this will be your first exposure to homeopathy. Perhaps you will find homeopathic medicine to be truly remarkable and will know that it is right for you. Or you may find homeopathic concepts intriguing but, for whatever reason, may not feel that this is the time or place to try them. I ask, as you read this book, that you remain open-minded—open to the true stories of women who were healed, often dramatically, with homeopathy and open to trying homeopathy yourself. Whatever the circumstances may be of your health, your life, and your healing and learning journey, I wish you happiness and well-being.

PART ONE

Homeopathy and Women:
A Perfect Match

Healing the Whole Woman

You Are Far More Than the Sum of Your Body Parts

YOUR BODY

Perhaps your physical concerns disturb you the most. The annoying, incessant, or even unbearable discomfort of a chronic yeast infection. The intermittent, and sometimes exhausting, flood of blood due to excessive menstrual bleeding. The misery of morning sickness. The excruciating pain of a miscarriage or labor. Or the agonizing discomfort of recurrent bladder infections. It may seem, in such cases, that you just want your body to feel better . . . the pain to go away . . . the bleeding to stop . . . your baby to be born.

Whether the approach is conventional or alternative, the goal is to relieve your pain and suffering. In your moment of intense discomfort, you might give anything for a quick fix . . . a strong pill . . . the big guns . . . having the problem part removed. You probably want your suffering to be taken away as rapidly as possible and be forever eliminated.

YOUR MIND AND EMOTIONS

Physical symptoms rarely occur in a vacuum. As you will learn in this book, illnesses seldom occur just on the physical level. "But," you might ask, "what if I develop a bladder infection after unusually active or frequent sex? Isn't that cut-and-dried? Physical cause generating physical effect?" That may or may not be the case. If a homeopath explores more deeply, he or she is likely to find that some emotional stress or trauma occurred just before an illness began. "What about a flu?" you might ask. "Or some other contagious disease? I was just in the wrong place at the wrong time." Maybe, but even in acute illnesses, and occasionally with first-aid situations, a certain vulnerability or stress may have been present before the sickness began.

Not every woman has to deal with the trauma of honeymoon cystitis following a sexual relationship with a new partner. Nor does every individual who is exposed to a cold or flu or strep throat actually get it. The ground must be fertile for the seed of disease to be sown before you can become ill. If you are not susceptible, even if everyone around you becomes sick, you will remain symptom-free. Mental and emotional imbalances can be severe and obvious or more subtle. Many physical problems are the result of unexpressed, repressed, or deeply buried emotions.

YOUR SPIRIT

Many illnesses arise out of an emptiness of spirit, a profound feeling of disconnectedness, separation, and isolation from God or Divine love. This deep sense of loneliness may originate from the traumas of childhood, disappointments during one's adult life, losses, illnesses, addictions, and personal pains of one sort or another. Often, such a state of poverty of spirit precedes a serious physical illness. A feeling of entrapment, in turn, generates a terminal illness from which there truly is no way out. Our health and illnesses are often a metaphor for our lives, beliefs, dreams, and perceptions. The idea that body, mind, and spirit are intertwined is becoming more widely accepted, and homeopathy is one of the only forms of medicine that can integrate and heal all three gently yet powerfully.

Edith's Story

Edith was a sixty-five-year-old financial planner from Minneapolis who first consulted me for depression nearly five years ago.

"My family practice doctor heard about your work and referred me here. I'm desperate. Two years ago I came down with a terrible flu. I was so weak that my knees buckled and I couldn't even hold up my head. My doctor called it chronic fatigue syndrome. It took a year before I got my energy back. Two months ago it started all over again, which surprised me since I did receive a flu shot last fall.

"People would call me a recluse. No partner and no support from my immediate family. That leaves a giant hole in my life that I try to fill partly with cigarettes. I've smoked for fifty years. Each time I inhale, I try to fill the void. No matter what I try, part of me just doesn't want to stop smoking. That part of me wants to kill myself, but not with emphysema. You're my last chance for hope.

"My childhood was horrendous. At sixteen my mother became pregnant. It was obvious that she never, ever wanted me. When I turned twenty, she actually told me how she'd tried to abort me with a clothes hanger. I almost starved to death during my first week of life because her nipples were inverted and I couldn't seem to keep any formula down. I've been starving ever since.

"I don't remember my mother touching me as a child. Not even once. Or protecting me. I never felt she was my mother and she did not feel I was her daughter. When I was six, she'd leave me at all-night movies and lock me in the car while she drank herself into oblivion at the bar for hours. I've blocked out most of my childhood.

"I didn't belong anywhere. I was so withdrawn in high school . . . almost catatonic. I started out with ten strikes against me and I've spent my whole life pulling myself up. Two poor choices of husbands, a son who was difficult from day one. My depression was so bad. It felt as if someone put a black bag over my head. Suicide seemed like the best option. Antidepressants helped for a while. Now the fatigue and depression are back. I'm going downhill again."

Edith noticed that when she bent forward, she felt as if her heart was in a vise. She had a long history of transient ischemic attacks (mini-strokes). Never rested, she awoke in the morning just as tired as she was the night before. She also complained of urinary dribbling and incontinence and had a lifelong aversion to eating. Although she had two grown children and grandchildren, she had next to no contact with any of them.

This is the kind of profound emptiness and disconnection that I spoke about. It's no accident that Edith suffered from transient ischemic attacks. Her heart was broken—so shattered that life no longer seemed worth living.

Edith's health and happiness have improved significantly, with the help of homeopathic *Aurum metallicum* (gold), over the past five years. She felt dramatically better within five weeks of taking the first dose and has needed ten or so doses in all. Edith reestablished contact with her children, her heart condition has been stable, and her outlook on life is much more positive. When I talked to her quite recently, she estimated the overall improvement in her health and emotional state to be 80 percent. Edith's deep alienation from and disappointment by life could have resulted in her suicide or death due to heart failure. Instead, she has to a large extent been healed. She still works on letting go of her smoking and, by her admission, has a ways to go, but she recognizes where she was five years ago and how far she's come. Her recovery, which I believe is more impressive than any she could have achieved with antidepressants, is a tribute to the healing power of homeopathy. Edith's heart is now much healthier, inside and out.

HEALING ALL OF YOU

Homeopaths have very high standards for healing. It's not enough just to have one or two of your main physical symptoms improve. Let's say you go to your gynecologist complaining of abnormal menstrual periods. You are put on the birth control pill to regulate your cycles. You may not have had time to mention your recurrent migraines or your panic attacks. Or perhaps you didn't bother because you went to a women's specialist who only addressed your irregular periods. You might be satisfied that the pill now regulates your cycle; however, you still have all the rest of your symptoms and you no longer ovulate. Your gynecologist might be satisfied that your periods are back to normal. End of story. The rest of your problems are not addressed, but you are considered fixed.

Not so with homeopathy. All of your symptoms must be significantly better or, at least, clearly progressing in the direction of healing for a homeopath to be satisfied that the medicine is correct. A homeopath considers the following criteria to be bottom-line in defining healing:

• *A significant, lasting improvement in your physical symptoms*—Your symptoms, most or all of them, need to be definitely better over a period of time—not just for a few months or every other menstrual cycle, but consistently and over at least one year. Better, by my standards, means that the symptom is either gone or is at least 70 percent better in terms of its frequency, intensity, and duration. You should be able to endure the same kind and level of stress that may have triggered your symptoms in the past, without getting those symptoms back to the same degree as before, if at all.

• *Increased energy*—You should feel more vital, energetic, and full of life. You should have a renewed zest, feel better when you wake up in the morning, and be able to accomplish your day's activities without feeling exhausted.

• *Mental stability and clarity*—This means clear thinking and the ability to concentrate and complete tasks, make wise decisions, reason out problems, and be intellectually sharp; to feel a sense of mental calmness and well-being despite the normal stresses of life.

• *Emotional balance*—Emotional equilibrium means experiencing the full range of human emotions without being stuck in any one emotion. You recognize happiness, love, and compassion as well as irritability, fear, and impatience. Your emotions are sufficiently in balance so that you can care about other people rather than being absorbed only in your own self. You are happy a good part of the time and get along well with others.

- *Enhanced creativity*—It doesn't matter whether the talent that gives you joy is painting, interior decorating, directing a choir, raising puppies, baking delectable desserts, styling hair, planning skyscrapers, designing programs to spread economic wealth, or, as I read about recently, traveling around the world making funny balloon-head ornaments to lighten everyone's spirits. What does matter is that it gives you the sense of exhilaration that occurs when you create something that is truly your own.

- *A sense of purpose or mission*—One of the greatest motivators of a long, happy life is a sense of contribution—that you do something that is important to, and makes a difference in, the lives of others. If you can give to others in a special, meaningful way, it makes your existence worthwhile.

- *Connectedness with other people*—Having close and loving family and friends with whom you can share your happiest and most challenging times is part of a healthful, balanced life. Solitude, a rare and undervalued commodity in our society, can be wonderful, but there is nothing like sharing a genuine, heartfelt bond with another being.

- *Spiritual satisfaction*—I recently saw a patient who had been through tough times in her life. Raised a Catholic, she confided that no matter how difficult the trial, she never doubted for a moment that God loved her. This abiding faith carried her through many a dark, and even suicidal, moment. Even in her loneliest times, she engaged in regular conversations with God, which gave her the strength and sustenance to go on.

Regardless of how tough your life has been, no healing is complete unless you realize a fundamental sense of peace and contentment. It is vital to hold that hope and vision even in the seemingly worst moments. I recently read a heartwarming story about a courageous and generous woman who has been through some of the most dreadful situations imaginable.

Sarah Kahaloa, or Miss Sarah, as she is lovingly addressed, is a forty-three-year-old woman who was born in a tiny village in Hawaii and now resides in Seattle. Once, she was beaten brutally by her father with a metal pipe; her legs and spinal column were so severely damaged that doctors doubted she would ever walk again. A year's worth of physical therapy finally elicited a twitch in her legs and she was eventually able to get around again. As a teenager, Miss Sarah was raped. Her first two husbands beat her and the second one abused other family members as well. Miss Sarah conquered alcoholism, drug abuse, and kidney cancer, which killed her great-grandmother, grandmother, and aunt. She lost her mother to leukemia. As if this were not more than enough, next came a recurrence of her kidney cancer and a metastasis to her ovary, followed by a torturous regimen of radiation and chemotherapy.

Miss Sarah's response? In addition to working twenty hours a week at an art store, she volunteers another twenty hours a week as a support worker for AIDS and hospitalized cancer patients. Every Thanksgiving for the past ten years, Miss Sarah has opened the doors of her small, housing-project apartment to anyone and everyone who has nowhere else to go. She offers food, solace, and a safe haven from the outside world. The only conditions she imposes are no drugs, alcohol, swearing, or fighting.

When Miss Sarah isn't working, volunteering, or handing out free food on Thanksgiving Day, she is often found dancing in the Seattle rain. "It's all by the grace of God that I'm able to do any of this, that I'm able to get up in the morning. I'm so thankful just to be able to walk. I even like the rain, how it waters the Earth."[1] Now that's gratitude!

CHAPTER 2

Drugs, Surgery, or Hormones— What Is Your Pleasure?

What Conventional Medicine Has to Offer You

HIGH-TECH MEDICINE IS GREAT WHEN YOU NEED IT

If you have the misfortune to suffer an injury in a car accident, you will no doubt wish to be transported as quickly as possible to the local emergency room. You will want the most skilled technicians to carefully examine you, identify the sites of injury, and embark on the most effective intervention with no time lost. Surely, the same is true if you suddenly develop appendicitis or if your child contracts meningitis. These are potentially life-threatening situations.

Yet conventional medicine, advanced as it is, does not necessarily have all the answers, nor is it harmless. Despite its great strides, modern Western medicine is in some ways still in its infancy, with much to learn from more traditional methods of healing, including homeopathy. You still take your chances with high-tech medicine. Consider this recent report: "Study: 98,000 Deaths Each Year Are Linked to Medical Mistakes." The president of the W. K. Kellogg Foundation, who chaired the committee that compiled the report, concluded, "These stunningly high rates of medical errors, resulting in deaths, permanent disability, and unnecessary suffering, are simply unacceptable in a medical system that promises first to 'do no harm.'"[1]

What if you escape from your minor automobile accident with a nagging whiplash injury? Or what if the abdominal pain does not turn out to be appendicitis but is an anxiety reaction to a new job? Or perhaps your child has a fever of unknown origin that will not respond to antibiotics. In each of these cases, high-tech medicine may not be your best bet once the diagnosis has been clearly established. In each of these cases, there may be far safer and more natural options available to you.

IF ALL YOU HAVE IS A HAMMER . . .

You've probably heard the expression "If all you have is a hammer, then everything looks like a nail." Let's say you are forty-two years old and have suffered from excessive menstrual bleeding for the past three months and a pelvic ultrasound has confirmed a grapefruit-sized uterine fibroid (which is, by definition, nonmalignant except in very rare cases). What are you to do? If you go to a surgeon, he will likely recommend a hysterectomy. He may suggest that because you do not plan to have more children, because menopause is not far away, and because the excessive bleeding is unpredictable, uncomfortable, and a nuisance, a hysterectomy is the best option. And, since you'll be undergoing surgery anyway, consider having your ovaries removed at the same time to prevent future problems that might occur.

This physician may have good intentions, speaking from his professional experience and offering what he believes to be sound advice. But he is a surgeon. His specialty is cutting out parts of the body that don't work. Even if he agrees to buy you some time with a D & C (dilation and curettage, in which the uterine lining is scraped) or an endometrial ablation (removal of the lining of the uterus), he probably believes that a hysterectomy is the ultimate solution to your problem. And, if his wife or daughter were in your situation, that is also what he would likely recommend to them.

It may simply not occur to someone who takes care of women's problems by removing organs or parts of organs, that there are effective, nonsurgical approaches. And why should it when, from his point of view, surgery works so permanently and so well? Except, of course, for the scar tissue, limited range of motion due to adhesions, and postsurgical pain, not to mention the emotional scars, which may last for a lifetime.

A PILL FOR EVERY ILL

Modern medicine consists, to a large degree, of pharmaceutical drugs. Whether your complaint is a headache, a bladder infection, anxiety, or depression, you are encouraged to take a pill to relieve your ill. The focus is on immediate relief rather than on understanding what caused the problem to occur in the first place and trying to prevent a recurrence. The typical, rushed physician's appointment doesn't allow time to delve deeply into the *cause* of the problem, only time to offer what promises to be a quick fix.

Now, if pain is your complaint and a pill takes it away, you might be quite satisfied. You might not care in the least whether the pill comes from a natural or a synthetic source. You just want to feel better fast and get back to work or to play, whatever was on your agenda before your illness interrupted you. And, as a quick fix, the pills might work fine.

Two main problems are associated with drugs, though. The first is that they have side effects. Often the side effects can be worse than the original complaint. The second is that they don't get to the root of the problem, so the problem will likely reoccur in the future.

Take, for example, my patient, Anna, who responded beautifully to homeopathy for morning sickness. Three weeks after the birth of her beautiful baby girl, who happened to be her third child, her right breast became painful and was throbbing. The answer offered by her obstetrician for the mastitis: an antibiotic. Anna followed his recommendation, and the pain subsided over the next few days. But then the baby developed thrush (an oral fungal infection) and the mother suffered from a vaginal yeast infection. Both were direct results of the antibiotic treatment, which indiscriminately eliminated the bacteria that supposedly caused the mastitis as well as the healthy flora in the intestines of mother and baby. The obstetrician then prescribed Nystatin, an oral antifungal medication with potential side effects to the liver, and urged Anna to supplement her breast milk with a cow's milk formula. Within three days the infant developed gas.

At this point, Anna, having little to no desire to give her month-old bundle of joy still more drugs, called me to see how homeopathy could help. Feeling quite frustrated at the turn of events after she had been able to remain so healthy during her pregnancy, she was ready to go the natural route again. I questioned the wisdom of the Nystatin, especially since the baby had suffered neonatal jaundice and Nystatin can potentially be hard on the liver. Anna felt it was much safer to discontinue the drug for both herself and the baby, so I prescribed a homeopathic medicine for mother and child, recommended supplementing her breast milk with goat's milk (which has the enzymes closest to mother's milk) rather than cow's milk, and suggested oral acidophilus for Anna to replenish her normal intestinal flora and, I hoped, the baby's as well. Within two days, all of the symptoms were resolved for both mom and baby.

This example illustrates a situation in which a pill just wasn't the answer. Had Anna consulted me for her mastitis (which generally responds quickly and successfully to homeopathic treatment), she could have avoided the thrush, yeast infection, and gas that ensued. Once she embarked on the conventional route after the birth, she just forgot to call me. Next time, I don't think she will. In addition, had she received homeopathic treatment for the mastitis, the chances of a recurrence weeks later would have been much less, whereas that is not necessarily the case after antibiotics. So side effects and possible future recurrences are two good reasons to look beyond drugs for women's problems.

There may be times when you do choose to take prescription drugs for very good reasons. You are in charge of your healing. Honor whatever decisions you make. Communicate closely with your doctor so that you continue taking the medications only as long as necessary. In some cases, such as with thyroid supplementation, you may need to be on the drugs for the rest of your life. In many other conditions, natural therapies such as homeopathy can help you, under the guidance of your prescribing physician, to eliminate your medications.

SURGERY

Surgery is a fine art and, at the right time and place, is indispensable. But in many cases, surgery is avoidable. Thirty million people in the United States undergo surgery each year, 70 percent of them women.[2] It is estimated that 824,000 hysterectomies will be performed in 2005.[3] Besides losing the ability to bear more children and experiencing whatever other emotional distress may accompany the loss of her uterus, and possibly her ovaries, a woman adjusting to (a sometimes premature) menopause can undergo a real shock. In addition, it has been shown that women who underwent a hysterectomy at age thirty-five ran a sevenfold higher risk of heart attack or angina.[4] Surgery is something to consider carefully.

Very early in my practice, a woman came to me complaining of profuse uterine bleeding during and between her periods. On performing a speculum exam, I found a tennis ball–sized fibroid protruding beyond her cervix. Through a combination of homeopathic and naturopathic recommendations and some inner work to examine the underlying cause of the fibroid, she was able to reduce the fibroid by half over the next three months. Had she continued the process, it is possible that it would have shrunk completely; however, the bleeding, less profuse but still uncomfortable, and her inability to have sex with her husband were more than she was willing to tolerate for another three months. I accompanied her to surgery, the now golf ball–sized fibroid was removed, and she followed our postsurgical program. Now, ten years later, she has not developed a recurrence of the fibroid. This is an example in which a minor surgical intervention in addition to natural medicine was all that was needed. Surely, many gynecologists would have recommended a hysterectomy in this situation. I have treated dozens of other women for uterine fibroids, and all but three have successfully avoided surgery.

Yet another condition in which surgery is recommended, often repeatedly, is endometriosis. Although conventional medicine has no real answer for why the uterus proliferates tissue in places where it should not normally be—from areas in the uterus itself to the abdomen, rectum, or even the lung—surgery is considered the best solution. Drugs may be used first to imitate a state of premature menopause so that the growth of endometrial tissue can be arrested. In many cases, homeopathy can be highly effective in alleviating all the symptoms of endometriosis without the necessity of any additional medication or surgery whatsoever.

As a homeopath, here are my recommendations if you are considering surgery:

• Research your condition yourself to confirm whether surgery is the treatment of choice for your particular situation. The Internet is an excellent way to become well-informed overnight. If you need help interpreting the data, ask your doctor or a knowledgeable physician on the Internet who provides that service. Get a second opinion. And, if necessary, a third. Some surgeries are urgent, others are not. Your surgeon may be willing to give you three to six months, or even longer, to try homeopathy or another natural approach so that surgery can be avoided. While breast cancer might require immediate surgery, uterine fibroids rarely do.

If you do choose surgery, find a skilled surgeon who has a lot of experience and an excellent track record and reputation in treating your particular problem. When I chose a free-flap microsurgery reconstruction following my mastectomy, I was led to a surgeon who had a success rate of nearly 100 percent and who had trained with the foremost expert in her field. My surgery had a very positive outcome.

• Be informed as to the precise extent of the surgery you choose. If it is a hysterectomy, can your ovaries be spared? If half of your thyroid needs to be removed, can you save the other half? I strongly advise not having anything removed unless it is absolutely necessary. Most surgeries are irreversible.

• Use a pre- and postsurgery protocol, such as the one in this book, to promote rapid recovery and prevent or minimize scar tissue formation.

• Ask your surgeon exactly what you can expect after surgery. How long will you need to recover? Will there be any lasting or permanent side effects from the procedure? What type of exercise can enhance rapid healing and how soon after surgery can you begin?

• If additional surgery may be required at the same time because of the surgeon's findings, what do you want him or her to do?

• In the case of day surgery, make plans as to where you will go afterward and who will be with you. How will you deal with any surgical side effects? (I have had two outpatient surgeries. After the first, I felt quite nauseous during the ride home and threw up. The second time, the anesthesiologist explained that he routinely puts an antinausea medication in the IV to prevent the patient from feeling sick later. Although I like to avoid drugs whenever possible, the medication was a blessing and I experienced no nausea whatsoever.)

- Do everything you can to make the surgery go as smoothly as possible. Follow all of the presurgery recommendations and visualize your surgeon, your anesthesiologist, and the rest of the surgical team doing their jobs perfectly, leading to your successful recovery. I have found hypnosis and deep relaxation to effectively alleviate fears about surgery and hospitalization.

- If you have special music that you wish to have played during your surgery, don't hesitate to ask.

- Is there someone whom you wish to accompany you to surgery and to be there when you wake up?

- Make sure that you engage in an inner examination of what has caused the surgery to be necessary so that you eradicate any seeds of future similar problems. Surgery is not a substitute for inner healing.

- After surgery, allow yourself to receive support, to rest, and to heal deeply. Don't overdo it too quickly. I learned this the hard way. Three months after my breast surgery, I spent six solid hours doing heavy weeding in my garden. I suffered left shoulder pain for months afterward just because I jumped into doing too much, too soon.

THE HORMONE DILEMMA

Perhaps the most controversial aspect of conventional drug therapy among women today is hormone replacement. The debate has heated up considerably due to recent evidence, published in the *Journal of the American Medical Association,* that the breast cancer risk for women taking estrogen plus progestin is considerably higher than for estrogen alone, up to an 8 percent increased risk per year. These alarming results are prompting many physicians to recommend that women limit synthetic hormone use to three to four years, which curtails long-term protection against heart disease and osteoporosis.[5] The heart disease–prevention rationale, previously a compelling reason for synthetic hormone use, is also being brought into question. A recent study led by Dr. David Herrington of Wake Forest University Baptist Medical Center in Winston-Salem, North Carolina, studied 309 postmenopausal women with heart disease and found four years of synthetic estrogen to have no benefit in slowing the buildup of fatty deposits in the arteries, which are considered the major underlying cause of heart attacks.[6] This research backs up the surprising findings of the Heart and Estrogen-Progestin Replacement Study, completed in 1998, which found women taking this common combination of hormones to be at an equally great a risk for new heart attacks as women already diagnosed with heart disease.[7] These two studies challenge the commonly held medical wisdom that since heart disease is the number one killer of postmenopausal women, the benefits of synthetic hormone replacement outweigh the risks. A federally sponsored Women's Health Initiative, which is examining the effects of hormone replacement on more than 27,000 women ages fifty to seventy-nine, should shed further light on the subject, although the first results are five years away.[8]

The decision of whether or not to use synthetic or, for that matter, natural hormones *is not cut-and-dried,* but rather a complex and multifaceted choice. Whatever your decision, check out current research thoroughly and keep your decisions in your own hands rather than those of your doctor or your partner. Dealing with menopause is, in some ways, like giving birth to a baby. You can have it all thought out ahead of time, like a pregnant woman who spends nine months planning for a home birth but then gives up on her birth plan once she's transported for a cesarean. When you're in the throes of hot flashes that wake you four or five times a night or you suffer from next-to-no libido, synthetic hormones can seem a lot more palatable than when you were premenopausally determined to go the natural route.

Remember that synthetic hormones are *not* a given. Whatever peri- or post-menopausal symptoms you experience, there may well be a natural answer without the risks of estrogen replacement. If you have a history of any condition that could become exacerbated with additional estrogen (including uterine fibroids, fibrocystic breasts, and breast cancer), take a good, hard look at the pros and cons before making a decision. Once you are in the office of a pro-hormone-replacement gynecologist, your defenses might be down and you might be convinced of something you would not normally have chosen if you had all your wits about you.

Nancy's Story

I recently had a rather disturbing incident with Nancy, a patient whom I hadn't seen in five years. Now menopausal and newly married to Greg, she came with him to my office to get help for her diminished libido. I did not find out until after the appointment that it was Greg who prompted her to call me. I spent an hour with the two of them, discussing the ups and downs of synthetic and natural hormone replacement, homeopathy, dietary and lifestyle measures to support menopause, the various kinds of soy, natural suppositories to take care of vaginal dryness, and more. Nancy listened avidly, partly because of her extensive history of severe fibrocystic breast disease, with more than half a dozen aspiration biopsies, as well as having lost her mother to breast cancer. Much to her relief, she had experienced no problem with her breasts for the past several years. Greg seemed to want a guarantee that whatever she took would raise her sex drive.

At the end of the appointment, Nancy seemed quite enthused about trying natural progesterone cream in combination with homeopathy, but Greg continued to object that there was not enough proof that natural hormone replacement could raise libido. The rest of the information I offered apparently fell on his deaf ears. Given her susceptibility to large, painful benign breast lumps and her mother's breast cancer, this is a woman who should be careful about estrogen replacement, yet she is clearly headed down that road for the sake of keeping her husband happy. I sincerely hope that they lead a happy life together and that she remains healthy and cancer-free, no matter how high or low her sex drive.

It is *your* body, *your* health, and *your* future. Do what is right for *you*, regardless of what anyone else thinks. You will want to consider many factors, such as your body type and baseline of bone density; what your mother's menopausal experience was like; your risk of osteoporosis; your risk or past history of breast and uterine cancer; your predisposition to heart disease and Alzheimer's disease; and your diet, lifestyle, and willingness to follow an ongoing program of weight-bearing exercise. It makes a lot of sense to sit down with someone knowledgeable who can help you make your decision. Since the greatest amount of bone loss occurs in the year immediately following your last period, the pros and cons of hormone replacement are something you will want to weigh even before your periods stop. In fact, you should begin taking calcium long before (preferably from the time you are a young woman) and begin a weight-training program at least by the time you enter perimenopause, preferably earlier. The choices may seem confusing, and indeed they can be, but you have the wisdom, given the right information, to make the right decision at menopause and the flexibility to change your mind later if necessary.

If you are a young woman who is considering taking hormones in any form for any reason, I encourage you, especially, to carefully consider the long-term consequences and the viable alternatives. With decades ahead of you, you will want to do everything you can to avoid osteoporosis as well as the various gynecological cancers. You may even want to consider individually formulated hormone replacement depending on your circumstances and family medical history.

CHAPTER 3

Homeopathy—What It Is and How It Can Help You

A Safe and Effective Natural Approach

LIKE CURES LIKE

Homeopathy is a medical science and an art unlike any other form of healing in a number of ways. Let me start with a simple definition. *Homeo* is Greek for "like" or "similar" and *pathos* means "suffering." Literally, homeopathy means "similar suffering." Translation: The very same substance that can produce a particular set of symptoms if you take it over and over again, can relieve those exact or very similar symptoms if you suffer from them. This is in contrast to most conventional medicine, which is also referred to as *allopathic medicine.*

Allo means "different." The basis of conventional medicine is to use drugs that are not at all similar to the disease, but that fight against it (antibiotics, antifungals, anti-inflammatories).

A simple example of this *law of similars* is a bee sting. If you ever happened to have the misfortune to cross a mad bee, you will be unlikely to forget the symptoms of the sting: swelling, redness, heat, and burning or stinging pain. The homeopathic approach to treating your bee sting, rather than using a topical conventional medicine, would be to use a substance capable of *causing* those very same symptoms. That substance in homeopathy is *Apis mellifica,* which is made from a honeybee. If, in fact, you take a dose of *Apis* soon after you are stung, it is very likely that the pain and discomfort will be alleviated within minutes.

However, *Apis* is not only good for bee stings, but for many other conditions that have similar symptoms. Now, think again: swelling, redness, heat, and burning or stinging. What other conditions could mimic these symptoms? How about an acute allergic reaction in which your face becomes quite swollen, red, and hot? Or conjunctivitis, with very swollen and puffy eyelids? Arthritis, in which the joints are inflamed, swollen, hot, red, and painful. Or a bladder infection with burning pain every time you urinate and a feeling of swelling in the urethra? Each of these conditions shares these four symptoms and can respond quite well to homeopathic *Apis*.

HOMEOPATHY HAS BEEN AROUND FOR TWO HUNDRED YEARS

Homeopathy has a proven track record. The concept of like cures like dates back to the writings of Hippocrates in 400 B.C. The concept of a vital force, or energy principle, had its origins in ancient Chinese and Asian texts. Homeopathy is based on this concept, as are acupuncture; Chinese, Ayurvedic, and Tibetan medicine; and most other indigenous medical systems. However, it took Dr. Samuel Hahnemann, a brilliant and bombastic German physician in the 1800s, to integrate all of these ideas into a single system of medicine: homeopathy.

Hahnemann was disgruntled, to say the least, with the barbaric medicine of his day. So, fed up with bloodletting, purging, and the use of toxic substances such as mercury and arsenic, Hahnemann decided to retire from his medical practice and focus his attention on medical translation. Fluent in seven languages, this original and creative thinker began to explore medical textbooks with the determination of finding a single principle on which all healing was based. There must, Hahnemann reasoned, be identifiable causes for why people get sick in the first place; for why they, in chronic disease, remain ill; and for how they recover from illness. Certainly, he surmised, this was not a random process.

The other fundamental motivation that drove Hahnemann was to find a safer, gentler, more effective method of treatment so that people like George Washington need not suffer from bloodletting applied haphazardly and, in cases such as his, fatally. Familiar with natural medicine traditions from all over the world, Hahnemann set out to find a better way.

And so he did. Upon reading in the herbal texts that the bark of the Peruvian cinchona tree (from which quinine is extracted) cures malaria, Hahnemann asked himself, "How and why is this possible?" Dissatisfied with the explanation of the herbalist authors, he embarked on a systematic ingestion (called a *proving*) of the bark itself. Through his own carefully documented experiments, Hahnemann verified the principle of like cures like. The intermittent sweats, fevers, and weakness that he suffered after ingesting the bark mimicked the actual symptoms of malaria. Convinced that he had discovered a unifying principle of healing, Hahnemann, and subsequently his students, set about to prove many common natural substances. Each proving was meticulously recorded and forms the basis for the knowledge that homeopaths have today. Next, Hahnemann and his fellow physicians administered these substances to their patients, in homeopathic preparations. The results were so impressive that the word spread of a remarkable new medical art.

In 1810 Hahnemann wrote his famous *Organon of Medicine,* which introduced homeopathy to the rest of the world. Though he was considered a medical heretic in his own country, many renowned European artists, musicians, writers, and playwrights nevertheless flocked to Hahnemann and his colleagues. By the mid-1820s, homeopathy had spread throughout Europe and reached the United States. By the turn of the century, homeopathic medical schools, hospitals, nursing homes, and sanitariums flourished in this country. In fact, around 1900, one out of every five or six medical doctors was a homeopath.

In 1910, while homeopathy continued to enjoy increased success in Europe, it was nearly crushed in the United States—thanks, in large part, to the Flexner Report. Andrew Carnegie commissioned a group to evaluate all of the American medical schools; and, as it turned out, all of the homeopathic institutions (as well as the practice of midwifery) were downgraded, resulting in their loss of funding and eventual closure. With no further formal homeopathic medical training, the profession gradually ground to a halt, with lay study groups in private homes and an occasional course here and there being the only way one could receive any exposure whatsoever to homeopathy. It is amazing that homeopathic medicine survived at all in the United States from 1920 to 1970, but somehow, thanks to its small but determined number of proponents, it did.

In the late 1970s, everything changed. The back-to-the-land and health food movements sparked interest in all that was natural, including homeopathy. A particularly strong group of homeopathic students in the Bay Area happened upon George Vithoulkas, a dynamic engineer-turned-homeopath, who came to the United States just at the time that many, including myself, discovered homeopathy. The tide of American homeopathy shifted since that time: Homeopathy has enjoyed a renaissance in this country. The quality of postgraduate homeopathic training programs is much higher, though not yet rivaling that of programs in Europe. Homeopathic courses and practitioners are sprouting up all over the United States, and I hope that we will one day again have a homeopathic medical school and separate profession.

HOLISTIC MEDICINE AT ITS FINEST

The very essence of homeopathy is understanding and treating the whole person. Homeopathy espoused this idea way before the term *holistic* came into vogue. Except in treating first-aid situations or with certain minor acute illnesses, a homeopath always undertakes an extensive, in-depth interview in which she investigates everything she can about the person in front of her. Without knowing and understanding the whole person, it is impossible to prescribe a homeopathic medicine for a chronic illness. The mental and emotional symptoms are considered to be at least as important as the physical ones. The picture of each individual is unique: like a jigsaw puzzle that, when each and every piece is put together, looks only like you and no one else. Or it can be compared to a tapestry of interwoven threads and colors that is only recognizable when the weaving is complete.

Imagine that you went to your doctor complaining of irregular periods with heavy bleeding and that you also suffered from premenstrual migraines that laid you up in bed for a day each month—plus, you have had eczema and asthma from a very young age. What if your doctor told you that she could give you one single medicine that would alleviate each and every one of these symptoms? Not a birth control for your periods, pain medications for your headaches, hydrocortisone cream for the eczema, and an inhaler for the asthma. But *one* medicine, which happened to be safe and natural, to boot. Would you find that impossible? Too good to be true? That is exactly what homeopathy promises to deliver.

DIFFERENT WOMEN DESERVE DIFFERENT MEDICINES

One of the beautiful features of homeopathy is that you are treated as an individual. Since the work of art that is your life, health, experiences, and being is unlike that of other women who may even have similar health problems, it makes sense that the medicine that will stimulate your healing is also unlike what many other women need. Even if you had a twin sister, it is probable that you would be quite different in a number of ways. That is how you are viewed by a homeopath: as a unique human being with a special story to tell.

Over two thousand homeopathic medicines are available, and new ones are being proven on an ongoing basis. Only by exploring your particular symptoms until the picture reveals itself clearly can a homeopath then match those symptoms to the single substance in nature that is most similar. When that match is made correctly, you will feel noticeably, often dramatically, better on all levels. If the match is incorrect, generally you will feel nothing at all and will merely report no change whatsoever.

Everything, past and present, that reveals your specific nature is important to a homeopath: your symptoms, language, interests, concerns, dress, dreams, work, hobbies, relationships, eating and sleep habits, and temperature preferences. There is little, if anything, about you that will not pique her interest. At the end of one or several homeopathic interviews, you will have communicated enough, in many ways, about yourself, that the medicine you need will become evident. Once that match is made, healing is bound to occur.

LAVENDER TO LADY'S SLIPPER

Absolutely every substance in nature is a potential homeopathic medicine. The only limitation is the time, energy, and expense associated with testing each substance. When you consider that there are over six billion human inhabitants of our planet, each uniquely herself or himself, it is not surprising that so many different medicines can be of benefit to different individuals. Two main types of books can be found in a homeopath's library: *repertories* and *materia medicas*. A repertory, which may be a heavy volume of a thousand or more pages (or may occupy an equivalent number of megabytes on a homeopath's hard drive), lists most of the imaginable symptoms, physical, mental, and emotional, that a person may experience and all of the homeopathic medicines that have been shown to cure each symptom. A *materia medica* is categorized according to each medicine and consists of one to many pages describing everything that is known about that medicine, depending on how well-known or widely used it is. In addition to the natural habitat, characteristics, and chemical structure of each substance, a *materia medica* discusses all of the conditions or systems of the body that have been healed by that particular substance.

Understanding the nature and breadth of scope of each substance opens up the entire natural world to the homeopath. Take, for instance, one of the most common women's medicines in homeopathy: *Sepia*. Pages and pages were written about the effects of this medicine, which is made from the cuttlefish, a relative of the squid. And much common knowledge about *Sepia* exists. Even if you have never even heard of homeopathy, the word *sepia* will bring certain ideas to your mind. You will probably think of those sepia-toned, brownish pictures that are found in portrait museums or aging family photo albums. Somewhere in your memory bank, you probably have stored the fact that squids release a dark, inky, protective juice (also called Indian ink), much like a smoke screen, and, if you have a culinary bent, you might even have tasted a dark-colored pasta flavored with its ink.

Sepia is commonly known among homeopaths worldwide for helping women who have a wide variety of physical complaints, including menstrual and menopausal difficulties, infertility and miscarriages, postpartum depression, morning sickness, and too many others to mention. The most well-known picture of a woman needing this medicine is of an active, independent, exercise-loving woman who feels that her independence has been lost once she has a child. She is no longer free to do as she pleases, she begins to feel unfortunate and miserable, she loses all sexual attraction toward her partner, and she just wants to run away. The feeling is one of being stuck, of being forced to do something against her will. A woman in this state is likely to crave vigorous, aerobic-type exercise and dancing, which seem to stir her out of her apathy.

Similarly, over two thousand other medicines have been made into homeopathic medicines, each with their own indications. Lady's slipper *(Cypripedium)* can be helpful for amenorrhea (absence of periods) and vaginal irritation, and lavender is helpful for excessive bleeding from anywhere in the body, including the uterus (which, surprisingly, had not been proven until I did so in one of my homeopathic classes at the same time that another homeopath had the same idea in England).

ARE YOU AN ANIMAL, PLANT, OR MINERAL?

Most homeopathic medicines come from three kingdoms: animal, plant, or mineral. This fun and fascinating exploration of the world of homeopathy might give you some food for thought. Once you have identified your kingdom, then, if you seek treatment from a homeopath for a chronic condition, the challenge is to figure out the particular member of the family that, when made into a homeopathic medicine, can alleviate your symptoms.

Animal types tend to be flamboyant, engaging, and vivacious, and they love attention. Or, at least, they seek to be this way. It is important for them to be attractive, competitive, and at the top. This is logical, given that animals continually engage in a survival of the fittest for their very sustenance. Women who need animal medicines (of which *Sepia* is one example) often have a conflict between their wild, undominated, born-to-be-free side and their domesticated, controlled, tame aspect. When difficult situations arise, they might respond with jealousy, aggression, dominance, and territoriality. Quick, alert, and vigilant, they are on the lookout for others who might strike or attack. Women in this group can be very seductive (either in their waking or dreaming states) and enjoy high sexual energy. In extreme cases, animal-like women, if enraged, can strike out, bite, or even growl. Their dress can be revealing, so if you see a colleague decked out in her leopard-skin dress and alligator shoes, watch out!

Plant types are in a different world from animal types, so to speak. Soft, gentle, changeable, and flowing, they are typically kind, sweet, and may be (though are not necessarily) self-effacing. The main feature that defines women needing homeopathic plant medicines is their sensitivity. It could be sensitivity to insults or criticism, the beauty of nature, others' suffering, injustice, noises, smells, light, or whatever. Women in this group tend to be adaptable and tenderhearted and to favor pastel, flowery, or lacy garments. You won't be surprised to learn that plant women love nature, gardening, landscaping, arranging flowers, and anything to do with plants. They flourish best in a well-tended, watered, and fertilized garden with high to low light, depending on their nature. Don't be harsh with a plant-type woman because it may hurt her deeply.

Last, but not least, are *mineral types*. Very different from the other groups, these women thrive on structure and order. They like things to be neat, organized, under control, and to live by the book. Just like the minerals from which the medicines they need are made, they are solid, grounded, and earthy. In fact, they may admire rocks and gems, like to spend their free time hiking in the mountains or buying diamonds, and often choose careers such as banking, accounting, architecture, financial planning, drafting, and engineering. If you go into your homeopath's office with an extensive, meticulous list of your past and present concerns, each one enumerated according to month and year, chances are you are a mineral type, particularly if you prefer clothes with stripes, checks, plaids, and geometrical designs.

The kingdoms are just one of many fascinating ways that a homeopath uses to figure out the one medicine that will most benefit you.

WEAKER IS STRONGER AND LESS IS MORE

Another distinguishing and intriguing aspect of homeopathic medicines is how they are prepared. No other type of medicine is prepared in this way. The reason homeopathic medicines are so safe and nontoxic is that they are made by a process of serial dilution and *succussion* (shaking).

What exactly does this mean? In order to make the preparation of *Sepia* that I mentioned earlier, the original pharmacy started out with one cuttlefish. The inky juice of that animal was prepared, according to FDA (Food and Drug Administration) standards, into an alcohol-based tincture called a mother tincture. This mother tincture forms the basis of the dilutions to follow. There are two scales of dilution measurement: decimal (parts of ten) and centesimal (parts of one hundred). While health food stores often sell decimal preparations (beginning with 1X), homeopathic practitioners more commonly use the higher, or centesimal, doses (denoted by C, such as 30C or 200C). For a decimal solution, one part of the original substance is added to nine parts of alcohol or water, then shaken vigorously. For a centesimal dilution, the ratio is one to ninety-nine. Further dilutions are prepared in the same way. The most common strengths of dilution, called *potencies,* that I use in my practice are 200C or 1M, meaning that the one to ninety-nine dilution and shaking have been repeated 200 to 1,000 times.

The more dilute, the stronger the medicine and the longer the effect. In other words, if you buy a 6X homeopathic preparation in a health food store, you may need to take it four times a day to achieve the desired effect, whereas I may only need to prescribe one dose of a 1M preparation once or twice a year for my patient to remain symptom-free.

HOMEOPATHY IS DIFFERENT FROM HERBS AND OTHER FORMS OF NATURAL MEDICINE

There are lots of different methods of natural healing, such as herbs, Chinese medicine, Ayurveda, nutrition, aromatherapy, and hydrotherapy, and it is easy to confuse one with another. Homeopathy is a type of natural medicine that is unique; although it may sometimes by combined with other forms of alternative medicine, it stands alone. It is specifically what I have mentioned: the use of one substance from nature, prescribed on the basis of like cures like, to heal the whole person.

Following are other natural approaches *not* to be confused with homeopathy:

- *Naturopathic medicine*—Practiced by a naturopathic physician who has graduated from a four-year full-time naturopathic medical school. It uses a variety of natural methods, including diet, herbs, homeopathy, hydrotherapy, and physical medicine, to stimulate the body to heal itself.

- *Holistic medicine*—Practiced generally by medical or osteopathic doctors. Relies primarily on the use of nutritional supplements as well as herbs, chelation, and other methods prescribed on the basis of (often extensive) laboratory testing, including hair and stool analysis and allergy testing. Different supplements are usually prescribed for each organ system, such as an adrenal extract, digestive enzymes, and a thyroid supplement.

- *Herbal medicine*—Although many homeopathic medicines are made from plants, the preparation is entirely different and so are, often, the indications for use. For example, St. John's wort *(Hypericum perforatum)* is a well-known botanical antidepressant. Its homeopathic uses include puncture wounds, skin infections, nerve injuries, and tailbone pain during pregnancy or after childbirth, just to name a few.

- *Chinese medicine*—An ancient system of medicine using acupuncture, Chinese herbs, and other lifestyle and energetic techniques to bring the body into balance.

- *Ayurvedic medicine*—A five-thousand-year-old form of healing from India that uses an integrated system of diet, herbs, yoga, gems, cleansing practices, and spiritual exercises to balance the overall constitution.

- *Chiropractic medicine*—Depending on the scope of practice in their states, chiropractors may work mainly on the spine and musculoskeletal system to align and rebalance your body or may use a variety of natural therapies, including any or all of those mentioned previously.

SO HOW DOES HOMEOPATHY WORK?

Although homeopaths have found consistently for over two hundred years that these medicines can be extremely effective for patients with all kinds of complaints, the specific mechanism of how or why homeopathy works is not yet clear. Although this is not very different from our limited understanding of how many pharmaceutical drugs work, some skeptics in the medical and scientific arenas nevertheless argue that homeopathy can't possibly work. No matter how much research we present (and clearly more is needed), some people deny the plausibility of homeopathy de facto, regardless of any positive double-blind studies. And, I wonder, how can those who claim that homeopathy has no possible way of being effective because there is "nothing in it" also claim that the medicines are dangerous? They can't have it both ways.

A number of possible explanations exist for why homeopathy works. It is becoming increasingly evident that treatments such as homeopathy and Chinese medicine work on an energetic or informational, rather than just a physiological, level. Hahnemann's own explanation was that, because homeopathic medicines are similar in nature to the symptoms from which the person is suffering, they induce a temporary, artificial illness powerful enough to replace the original one. This medicinally-induced disease, Hahnemann explained, is shorter-acting and rapidly disappears, leaving the person well.[1]

More recently, the formation of liquid crystals has served as the basis for explaining the effectiveness of homeopathic microdoses. Such crystals, it is suggested, facilitate the memory of water for what was contained in the original, diluted material. This line of research hypothesizes that water, the most common medium for homeopathic medicines, is capable of storing the memory of antigens and of facilitating physiological and immunological changes at the cellular level using dilution levels at which no chemical substance should remain.[2]

And so the mystery of the microdose remains until a time comes when the answer is revealed. In the meantime, until we can accumulate sufficiently extensive research to convince the doubters, homeopaths rely on the anecdotal stories, such as those in this book, of patients who have responded well to homeopathy. One of the most convincing demonstrations of the effectiveness of homeopathy is in videotapes of patients (who have, of course, given their permission) before and after their homeopathic treatment. When a naysayer argues that homeopathy couldn't possibly work because we don't understand its mechanism, I reply, "I invite you to sit in my office for a day, listen to the stories of my patients, and then tell me homeopathy doesn't work." Ironically, many of the greatest supporters of homeopathy were those who originally set out to disprove it.

Additional references from the scientific literature on homeopathic research are included in the notes.[3]

THE FLOURISHING OF HOMEOPATHY AROUND THE WORLD

Homeopathy is a household word in many parts of the world, from western Europe to India to South America. If you visit France, for example, and wander into one of the more than 22,000 pharmacies, you will find homeopathic medicines just as available as conventional over-the-counter medications. This is because most French pharmacists are trained in homeopathic pharmacology, and homeopathic medicines are fully reimbursed by the national health-care system. Thirty-six percent of the French population has sought out homeopathic treatment.[4]

Homeopathy enjoys similar widespread acceptance in Great Britain, where approximately 42 percent of family practitioners refer patients to homeopathic practitioners, many of whom are likewise covered by national health care. Nearly 10 percent of German doctors specialize in homeopathy and an additional 10 percent prescribe homeopathic medicines in addition to the 11,000 *Heilpraktikers* who use homeopathy and other forms of natural medicine.[5] Mexico, Argentina, and Brazil are also centers of widespread homeopathic practice.

The British carried homeopathy with them to India, where it spread like wildfire due primarily to its philosophy, accessibility, and affordability. There are now over 120 homeopathic medical colleges in India. Some of the best homeopathy in the world is practiced in India, which is why my husband and I study regularly with our mentors from Bombay.

The United States is at the forefront of natural medicine in many areas but still lags behind in its acceptance of homeopathy, due perhaps in part to the limited, though growing, number of experienced homeopathic practitioners.

WHO PRACTICES HOMEOPATHY IN THE UNITED STATES?

The number of homeopathic practitioners in this country is estimated to be around a thousand; however, the amount of interest and number of students are mushrooming. Since there is no licensing for homeopathic medicine, per se, practitioners either practice under the scope of their other medical licenses or are unlicensed. The largest number of medically trained homeopaths are either naturopathic physicians (N.D.) or medical doctors (M.D.); however, there are osteopaths (D.O.), chiropractors (D.C.), physician assistants (P.A.), nurse practitioners (N.P. or F.N.P), acupuncturists (L.Ac.), dentists (D.D.S.), and veterinarians (D.V.M.) taking up the practice of homeopathy. Since the medicines themselves are FDA-regulated, these practitioners with medical licenses of one sort or another operate under the scope of practice of their license in their particular state and may use homeopathy in part or all of their practice. Board certification is available to naturopathic doctors through the Homeopathic Academy of Naturopathic Physicians (D.H.A.N.P. certification) and medical and osteopathic doctors through the American Institute of Homeopathy (D.Ht.). In addition, many unlicensed homeopathic practitioners take a certification exam to demonstrate competence but do not have formal medical training or licensure.

The practice of homeopathy varies widely in this country. What we refer to in this book is *classical homeopathy,* which entails an interview of at least one hour in which the practitioner mostly listens to the patient, then asks some questions, and prescribes a single homeopathic medicine in one or more doses. Usually, there is an interim period of at least four to six weeks between appointments. The medicine is selected on the basis of the information provided in the interview rather than by muscle testing, pendulum, or machine. One single medicine, rather than a combination formula, is always prescribed by a classical homeopath.

My husband and I, and certain other homeopaths, enjoy treating patients by phone when there is no experienced, local homeopathic practitioner in the area where the patient lives. What is most important, when you select a homeopath, is determining that:

- he or she practices classical homeopathy
- he or she is board-certified, if that is available in his or her profession
- he or she has at least five hundred hours (minimum) of postgraduate training in classical homeopathy
- the initial appointment lasts at least one hour (often one and a half or two hours)
- the effect of each medicine is generally not evaluated any sooner than four to five weeks after it is administered (when treating chronic illness)
- the homeopath engages in ongoing continuing education (the current learning curve is extremely high and a wealth of new information becomes available each year)
- at least 50 percent of his or her practice (and, it is hoped, over 75 percent) is devoted to homeopathy
- he or she preferably has a minimum of five years in practice, especially in complex or serious cases (although this is not always possible and there are less-experienced practitioners who are very knowledgeable)

Please consult the appendix for further information on homeopathic resources.

CHAPTER 4

Why Many Women Choose Homeopathy over Conventional Medicine

Compelling Reasons to Make Homeopathy Your Medicine of Choice

HOMEOPATHY TREATS WOMEN, NOT DIAGNOSES

Homeopathy is very different from conventional medicine in a number of significant ways. First, a homeopath views you as a one-of-a-kind woman, takes into consideration all that is going on with you as a whole person, and selects one medicine to treat all of you, not just your particular complaint.

Second, homeopathic medicine has a different philosophy of why you may fall ill in the first place. It is inevitably due to an imbalance in your overall energy system. Simply said, if you are in complete balance, no matter what you are exposed to or how stressful your life, you will not become sick. If you are out of balance, you will. Take, for instance, a candida infection of the vagina, commonly known as a yeast infection. If your flora, tissue, and organism are healthy, there will be no breeding ground for such an infection to develop. If you lack lactobacilli (the friendly bacteria that reside in your colon or vagina), perhaps due to a recent regimen of antibiotics, the ground will be fertile for infection. However, regardless of the type of bacteria, fungus, or illness, the ultimate cause, according to homeopathic thinking, is *always* an imbalance in your energy system (vital force). This is much like Chinese medicine, which affirms that the *chi* or *ki* must be in balance and flowing harmoniously through the meridians of your body in order for you to remain healthy.

Third, homeopathy very much brings into balance the mental and emotional sphere, as well as the physical. It is very common among some women, for example, to suffer bladder infections after they have suppressed their anger. If this is true of you, take antibiotics as many times as you want, but it is unlikely that you will eliminate your tendency to develop bladder infections entirely until you address the cause: the stuffed emotions. You could try an approach of using psychotherapy, hypnosis, or another mind–body exploration to get to the root of the anger. Or you could take a homeopathic medicine—in this case, possibly *Staphysagria* (stavesacre)—which would, over time, allow you to feel and express your anger more freely, as well as eliminate the symptoms of the bladder infection and any other symptoms that you might have or develop.

HOW LIKELY IS HOMEOPATHY TO HELP YOU WITH YOUR SPECIFIC PROBLEM?

With the understanding in mind that homeopathy treats women as whole beings—mind, body, and emotions—and, specifically, brings the vital force into equilibrium, the following are chronic women's conditions that can benefit from homeopathic treatment. I have grouped them into five categories: those that have an *excellent* chance of being healed by treatment with a homeopath, those that *frequently* respond to homeopathy, those that are more challenging but *may* respond to homeopathic treatment so that it is worth a try (the "What have you got to lose?" category), conditions that respond best to a *combination* of homeopathy and other therapies, and those that have such a small likelihood of healing from homeopathy that it is best to *try another approach*. I've included in the list problems covered in this book. Homeopathy can be extremely effective with all kinds of other physical, mental, and emotional conditions as well.

Excellent Response to Homeopathy

Abnormal menstrual bleeding
Anxiety
Bladder infections (recurrent)
Depression
Endometriosis
Fatigue
Gall bladder problems
Headaches
Heavy periods (menorrhagia)
Irregular periods

Menopause

Menstrual pain (chronic dysmenorrhea)

Mood swings

PMS

Postpartum depression

Pregnancy

Vaginal infections

Frequent Response to Homeopathy

Acne rosacea

Eating disorders

Herpes

Human papilloma virus (HPV)

Low sexual energy

Urinary incontinence

Venereal warts

May Respond to Homeopathy

Absence of periods (Amenorrhea)

Infertility

Miscarriages (recurrent)

Ovarian cysts

Pelvic inflammatory disease

Polycystic ovaries

Respond Best to Homeopathy Combined with Other Therapies

Acne vulgaris

Anemia

Breast cancer

Cervical dysplasia

Osteoporosis

Sexual abuse

Uterine fibroids

Vaginismus

Better to Try a Different Approach

Ovarian cancer

Uterine cancer

Weight problems

SAFE, NATURAL, NONTOXIC

- All homeopathic medicines are carefully regulated by the FDA and prepared by high-quality homeopathic pharmacies.
- Homeopathic medicines are diluted repeatedly to the point that no remaining molecule, but only the pattern or imprint of the original substance, remains. Therefore, you do not have to worry about side effects, even for pregnant women, newborns, and the elderly. No *PDR (Physicians Desk Reference)* is needed for homeopathic medicines. Even infants could swallow an entire bottle of homeopathic pills with no harmful effects.
- Homeopathic medicines are made from natural substances from the plant, animal, and mineral kingdoms.
- In cases in which animals are used to make a homeopathic medicine, usually little or no injury is done to the animal. The same honeybee that was used by one homeopathic pharmacy has served to make millions of homeopathic preparations of *Apis mellifica*. In most cases it is the milk or venoms of a particular animal that is used in homeopathic provings.
- Homeopathic medicines cannot trigger allergic reactions.
- The medicines are so gentle and subtle that they cannot interfere with your prescription medicines.

If you ever do have an oversensitive reaction to a homeopathic medicine, which is rare, consult a homeopathic practitioner.

INDIVIDUALIZED TREATMENT

- You will be listened to and treated as a unique individual.
- You will be given one of over two thousand homeopathic medicines, so if one is not effective, another generally will be.
- Your homeopath will take into account all that has happened to you from birth through adulthood, in an attempt to discover the thread that runs through your case.
- Homeopathy seeks to understand what makes you different from every other person, rather than fit you into a diagnostic box.

TREATS ALL OF YOUR SYMPTOMS AT ONCE

- Homeopathy takes into account your whole being: every significant symptom, pattern, dream, fear, and trait.
- A homeopath will see you as a whole person rather than as a breast or an ovary.
- If you take the correct homeopathic medicine, not one, but all of your symptoms will generally improve.

- You will not need to see one homeopath for your joints, another for your skin, and a third for your gynecological problems. Homeopaths are general practitioners, taking all of you into account, even if they have a particular specialty other than homeopathy.
- You will need only one medicine, not a medicine chest full of prescription medications or a cupboard full of vitamins and minerals (though taking a reasonable number of supplements supportively is recommended).

MENTAL AND EMOTIONAL AS WELL AS PHYSICAL HEALING

- Homeopathy by definition will bring about mental and emotional as well as physical well-being. Not only your physical health, but also your mental clarity, attitude, emotional balance, and enthusiasm for life will improve.
- The mind and body are inextricably intertwined and treated as one whole organism in homeopathy. You could no more separate them than you could cut off your head from your body and still survive.
- Homeopathy can help you release emotions that you have carried with you for years.
- It is possible through homeopathy to let go of dysfunctional familial patterns that originated even before you were born.
- Being treated homeopathically prior to your pregnancy or the birth of your child can improve significantly the mental and emotional state of your child.
- You can experience mental and emotional well-being without the disturbing side effects of psychiatric medications.

ADDRESSES THE ROOT OF THE PROBLEM

- The homeopathic interview process is extensive and in-depth. A good homeopath will continue the interview until she has really grasped the thread that ties together all of your symptoms: physical, mental, and emotional.
- You might gain considerable insight into your problem just from the initial homeopathic interview, even before you take the medicine.
- The subconscious mind, in the form of dreams, carries great importance in homeopathy as a key to unlocking underlying motivations, patterns, and hindrances.
- If you are already seeing a psychotherapist, once the correct homeopathic medicine is given, your progress in therapy may be enhanced and proceed more quickly.
- After you take the correct medicine, a shift takes place within you that, over a period of months or years, can produce significant, often dramatic, positive changes.

- As you undergo effective homeopathic treatment, even your dreams can change in content and feeling, signaling a transformation on the subconscious as well as the conscious level.

CURATIVE RATHER THAN SUPPRESSIVE

- Homeopathy does not seek Band-Aid or partial improvement. In order for a homeopath to be convinced that the medicine is correct, *all* of you must be better, not merely certain parts of your body at the expense of other parts.
- Whatever you have suppressed in the past, be it a skin eruption or your anger, often comes out in the process of homeopathic cure. Since homeopathic medicines are quite gentle, this usually occurs over a period of time.
- You do not have to worry that homeopathy will dampen healthy emotional expression. If, for instance, you experience significant grief after the death of a parent, homeopathy will allow you to grieve fully and then move on. It will not rob you of the emotional experience that you need to learn and to grow.
- If you are in a relationship, job, or other situation that is unhealthful and causes you to suppress your individuality, creativity, opinions, or freedom of choice, you may find yourself, sometime during the course of homeopathy, either releasing the situation or doing whatever is necessary to resolve it and be yourself.
- Homeopathy will not prolong life or suffering unnaturally, although, when given to a dying patient, it can ease the transition.

PRODUCES LONG-LASTING, OFTEN PERMANENT, CHANGE

- Homeopathy is *not* a quick fix, but is instead an ongoing process that, over time, increases health, balance, and well-being.
- A single dose of a homeopathic medicine may last for months or years, rather than just a few hours like most conventional medicines.
- Homeopathic medicines have a cumulative effect. They do not work on only a physiological basis, and their effects become stronger and more stable over time.
- You may find that after two or three years of homeopathic treatment you feel so well and so permanently changed that you see your practitioner only for an occasional acute illness.

HOMEOPATHIC MEDICINES ARE VERY INEXPENSIVE

- A lifetime supply of your homeopathic medicine often costs less than a single month's worth of your prescription medicine.

- Less is more with homeopathy, so you only take the medicine when you need it, which is generally not very often.
- Homeopathic medicines have no expiration date, so they will last forever unless they run out.

PROTECTION AGAINST FUTURE ILLNESS

- By bringing the vital force into balance, homeopathy automatically strengthens the immune system.
- In the eyes of a homeopath, your best protection against future illness is to receive the correct homeopathic medicine for you as a whole person (called *constitutional treatment*).
- Women who use homeopathy regularly often report that they and their children (if also treated homeopathically) get fewer acute illnesses like colds and the flu.
- Homeopathy increases stamina and vitality.
- If you are treated homeopathically prior to conception or giving birth to your child, it may increase the baby's protection against serious illness.

AN EFFECTIVE ALTERNATIVE TO DRUGS OR SURGERY

- Women who seek out homeopathic treatment for their health problems prior to taking prescription pharmaceuticals often find that they no longer need to take them.
- If you are already taking medication for your condition and are interested in being able to discontinue it in the future, homeopathy can often help you do that, under the guidance of your prescribing physician.
- If you worry about the side effects of taking your medications long term, or about the possibly damaging effects on your unborn child, or if you think you take entirely too many different prescription medications, homeopathy might be the right course for you.
- Homeopathy can make surgery for such conditions as uterine fibroids, ovarian cysts, and many others problems unnecessary.

HOW TO DECIDE WHETHER HOMEOPATHY IS RIGHT FOR YOU

Constitutional homeopathy is a commitment of time, energy, money, and hope that is extremely worthwhile for a large number of women. You are the only one who can decide whether it is the right step for you. You may be convinced, after reading this book, that homeopathy sounds like just what you need. If you're not sure, you can try homeopathic self-care if your condition is suitable. You may want to investigate through further reading or talking to others who have tried homeopathy. I see, on a daily basis, the profound transformation and healing that homeopathy can bring when the timing is right, the patient is willing and ready, and the homeopath finds the best medicine to bring about a deep and lasting cure.

CHAPTER 5

How Homeopathy and Conventional Medicine Can Work Hand in Hand

A Compatible Relationship If Both Partners Are Willing

HOMEOPATHY DOES NOT INTERFERE WITH CONVENTIONAL MEDICATIONS

You or your doctor may be concerned about homeopathic medicines interfering in some way with your conventional treatment. Simply put, this will not happen. In comparison to pharmaceutical drugs, homeopathic medicines are very safe and gentle. If anything, the effects of strong prescription medications may overpower the effects of the more subtle homeopathic preparations, but not vice versa. But they can often work effectively, side by side. If you choose to continue taking your conventional medications, homeopathy can give you more energy, relieve physical complaints that your medicines do not touch, improve your clarity of mind and emotional balance, and enhance your overall sense of well-being. In no way can they undo the effectiveness of your prescribed medications.

I'M NOT SURE IF HOMEOPATHY IS FOR ME—HOW CAN I FIND OUT?

Let's say you are somewhat, but not extremely, dissatisfied with the drugs that you take; however, you are curious about a more natural alternative. Can you somehow stick your toes in the water without taking the entire plunge? Sure. You may want to try one of the following approaches.

- **One step at a time:** Continue seeing your conventional doctor but try treating yourself for acute conditions such as vaginitis, mastitis, and acute bladder infections. You don't have to change health-care practitioners, stop taking any medications, make any lifestyle changes, or commit yourself to a new form of healing. Just try it out and see how it works for you.

- **Straddle the fence:** If you're not entirely happy with the health care you currently receive, consider establishing a relationship with an experienced homeopathic practitioner. In most cases, you can continue the conventional protocols that you already follow and see your regular doctor or practitioner in addition to the homeopath. If you find that homeopathy works very well for you, it is usually possible to discontinue your conventional medications (hopefully with the blessing and guidance of the prescribing physician). You may find that you like homeopathy so much that it becomes your medicine of choice, both for acute and chronic problems.

Two situations in which I commonly see women combining what both have to offer are menopause and breast cancer. Many women take hormone-replacement treatment with mixed emotions. If they could find a natural alternative that would make their hot flashes go away or even tolerable, lubricate their vaginal tissue, help them remain happy and healthy, and prevent osteoporosis and heart disease, they would toss the hormones in a heartbeat. Women undergoing surgery, chemotherapy, and/or radiation for breast cancer are, more and more, looking for adjunctive natural therapies to stay healthy amid the onslaught of powerful and toxic treatments.

No one says that you must choose *either* homeopathy *or* conventional medicine. One exception is if you wish to be treated for hormonal problems and you are taking birth control pills. Since you will no longer ovulate and all or most of your hormonally related symptoms will be gone or masked, your homeopath might ask you, as I do, to stop the pill before beginning homeopathic treatment.

If you ultimately decide to choose homeopathy as your primary source of health care, you can still use conventional medicine as a backup for emergencies, diagnostic procedures, and more invasive procedures if they are needed.

CONVENTIONAL MEDICINE IS NOT FOR ME— CAN I USE HOMEOPATHY INSTEAD?

In many cases, the answer is yes. Although in certain areas conventional, high-technology medicine has a great deal to offer, in others you may have reached the limits of its expertise. Or you may simply want to try a safer and more natural kind of treatment for a year or two before submitting yourself to an invasive approach.

In this book you will read a number of autobiographical stories by women who have found great relief from homeopathy for their gynecological problems and who seek out the care of their homeopath before even considering more drastic procedures. Once you have a correct diagnosis, as long as your condition is not urgent or life-threatening, there is no reason why you should not choose homeopathic treatment, as long as you can find an experienced and qualified practitioner whom you trust.

Two situations in which I have seen this occur repeatedly are with endometriosis illnesses and during pregnancy. As I elaborate on in chapter 13, the conventional treatment for endometriosis, which includes hormones and surgery (often more than one), is not only invasive and traumatic, it is often ineffective. Women who have already undergone this regimen with little or no success are frequently thrilled to find a gentle, natural alternative.

Women suffering from all kinds of problems during pregnancy may be understandably resistant to taking drugs that could harm their unborn child. This is an area in which homeopathy can provide tremendous benefits since most health problems, physical, mental, and emotional, of pregnant women can be addressed beautifully with homeopathy, with absolutely no danger whatsoever to the fetus.

CAN I USE MY HOMEOPATH AS MY PRIMARY-CARE PRACTITIONER?

Often you can. You need to have someone, be it your homeopath (if so qualified) or another physician or practitioner, who can correctly diagnose any medical problems that might arise. This will alleviate any concern that your homeopath might miss a diagnosis. In actual fact, your homeopath, because she spends so much more time listening to your concerns, might even catch a diagnosis that your conventional doctor has missed.

Many women are so overjoyed with the benefits of homeopathy that they prefer to use it as their treatment of choice whenever possible—which, in my experience, is much of the time with both acute and chronic illnesses. Some exceptions are emergency situations such as injuries, ectopic pregnancies, appendicitis, severe pneumonia, blood poisoning, heart attacks, and strokes. Even in some of these cases, homeopathic medicines can speed up healing and recovery if used in conjunction with conventional medicine.

If you do choose your homeopath as your primary-care practitioner, she will provide you with guidelines for when to contact her first and when to seek out emergency or conventional care before contacting her. Some homeopathic physicians carry pagers so they can be readily reached in case of emergency, and they are willing to provide adjunctive care if you find yourself hospitalized. What is most important is that you work out a system of health care in which you have confidence and can rest assured that your needs will be met.

SUPPRESSION VERSUS CURE

Suppression means the removal of a symptom or group of symptoms without addressing the underlying cause. Imagine that you had a hysterectomy as a solution for excessive menstrual bleeding. You might say that your problem is fixed because your uterus was responsible for the bleeding and now it is gone. But homeopathy would offer a different explanation and solution. Why were you bleeding abnormally in the first place? There was an imbalance in the vital force, your genitourinary system was the area of weakness, and that imbalance expressed itself through excessive bleeding. It is entirely possible that you experienced an emotional trauma just before the bleeding began, which triggered a physical response. Or you may have a predisposition to exaggerated bleeding in other areas of your body as well, such as recurrent nosebleeds. A hysterectomy would certainly not correct that underlying tendency, whereas homeopathy would.

Most conventional medicine approaches disease through suppression. Your nosebleeds, if persistent, might be addressed through cauterization or even surgery. Bladder infections are treated with antibiotics; venereal warts with strong, topical applications or laser surgery; yeast infections with antifungal preparations; acne vulgaris with topical or oral antibiotics or retinoic acid; and cancer with surgery, radiation, and/or chemotherapy. Conventional medicine does not attempt to work *with* the body to alleviate disease; the goal, rather, is to eradicate the symptoms.

In many cases, suppressive therapies do seem to remove the offending symptom(s), sometimes temporarily, sometimes permanently. However, the original symptom may disappear only to be replaced by a second, more serious one. A classic example is the treatment of infantile eczema with hydrocortisone cream. There is little or no attempt to understand *why* that child is manifesting eczema, an allergic condition, in the first place. It might be a simple case of the mother introducing cow's milk into the child's diet too early, which could be remedied simply by feeding the baby only mother's milk and/or goat's milk. Assuming only topical hydrocortisone is used, homeopaths commonly see a progression from eczema, a relatively mild though annoying condition, to asthma, another allergic condition that is much more severe and potentially life-threatening. This is an example of suppression. The eczematous itching is now replaced by wheezing and shortness of breath, and now bronchodilators or, often, corticosteroids are the drugs of choice.

Some people are more prone to suppression than others. One area in which I have seen this phenomenon occur in a worrisome way in women is with tumors. You might be a woman who has a predisposition to growths. These growths could be as innocuous as pimples, moles, or warts that could appear anywhere in or on your body. A bit more bothersome are lipomas (fatty deposits), sebaceous cysts, or cervical polyps. Or you might suffer the discomfort of fibrocystic breast disease, a benign, cystic type of growth.

At this stage, although they are not serious, your doctor might recommend surgery. You may notice that even if one of these growths is removed, another comes in its place. Your vital force, or energy system, has for some reason an inclination to create growths. If you continue to remove them without examining and eliminating the cause, your body will continue to have the same tendency and may eventually, if all of its other outlets are removed, try to generate more serious growths such as uterine fibroids, ovarian cysts, or even malignant tumors. Some women, depending on their constitutions, are more likely to suffer harmful repercussions from suppression than others.

CONVENTIONAL MEDICATIONS FOR WOMEN'S CONDITIONS THAT ARE COMPATIBLE WITH HOMEOPATHIC TREATMENT

The following types of commonly used drugs, in my experience, rarely interfere with homeopathic treatment. However, with effective homeopathic treatment, you may no longer need them if your problems are resolved.

antacids	bronchodilators
anti-anxiety medications	decongestants
antidepressants	diuretics
antihistamines	hormone-replacement therapy
anti-inflammatories	pain relievers
beta-blockers	sleep medications
blood pressure medications	thyroid medications

CONVENTIONAL MEDICATIONS THAT CAN INTERFERE WITH HOMEOPATHIC TREATMENT

Some conventional medicines stand a greater chance of masking or suppressing symptoms to the point where your homeopathic treatment may be confused, obstructed, or ineffective. They include:

antibiotics	chemotherapy
antifungals	corticosteroids (oral or topical)
birth control pills	narcotic drugs

In order to optimize the success of homeopathic treatment when you're taking these medications, your homeopath may postpone starting treatment, suggest another option instead of homeopathy, ask you to talk to the prescribing physician about discontinuing or decreasing the dosage of your conventional drugs (if appropriate), or administer the homeopathic medicine more frequently.

Antibiotics sometimes, but not always, interrupt homeopathic treatment. In many cases, the correct homeopathic medicine or herbs can be used instead to effectively alleviate infections. Birth control pills generally do prevent pregnancy, but, because they also stop ovulation and mask or eliminate gynecological symptoms, they are the

Enlist the Support of Your Conventional Health-Care Practitioner for Homeopathic Care

Below are tips for enlisting the support of your doctor for your use of homeopathic treatment.

- The more you come across as a reasonable, self-directed, and well-informed patient, the more likely your doctor is to respect your decisions and point of view.

- If you wish to share with your practitioner that you are using homeopathy, do so openly and honestly.

- If your doctor says there is no scientific corroboration of homeopathy or that it is only a placebo, inform her that over one hundred studies have been conducted, including some favorable ones published in highly respected medical journals.

- If you feel intimidated by your doctor and cannot share your opinions, either take an advocate with you or find someone with whom you can feel at ease.

- If your doctor is afraid that homeopathic medicines can interfere with conventional drugs, assure him that this is not the case.

- If you are told that you have no time to try an alternative treatment, ask the doctor why and, if necessary, get a second opinion.

- If your doctor categorically opposes alternatives and threatens to stop seeing you if you choose them, it may be time to find a more open-minded and tolerant doctor.

- If your practitioner is confused about what homeopathy is or seems genuinely interested in homeopathy, ask her if she would like to learn more about it, and suggest resources.

- If your physician is concerned about side effects, explain that homeopathic medicines are nontoxic and safe even for newborns and pregnant women.

- Ask your practitioner to remain open-minded and encouraging about your response to homeopathic treatment.

- When homeopathy works well, share the results with your doctor so he can be better-informed and can learn that homeopathy is effective.

least natural of birth control methods. If you seek homeopathic help for women's problems, it may be best to switch to another form of birth control first, such as a cervical cap, condoms and foam, or a diaphragm. Narcotic drugs, whether used for pain or for recreational purposes, are very powerful and addictive and can potentially interfere with homeopathy. Corticosteroid preparations, whether topical hydrocortisone, oral Prednisone, or a steroidal inhaler or nasal spray, dampen the natural immune response and are some of the most suppressive drugs. They may be necessary at times but can have severe side effects as well as being difficult to discontinue. You may, however, be able to gradually taper off steroid use, under your doctor's care, once your homeopathic treatment has begun to work. Chemotherapy, because of its toxicity, may necessitate the use of more frequent administrations of your constitutional homeopathic medicine, as well as additional ones to lessen the nausea, weakness, and other often debilitating side effects.

CHAPTER 6

When to Treat Yourself and When You Need a Homeopath

FIRST AID, ACUTE, OR CHRONIC?

Homeopathy, in the hands of a skilled practitioner treating *chronic* conditions, is elegant yet very complex. Self-treatment for *first-aid* and *acute* conditions, on the other hand, can be remarkably simple and require very little knowledge to achieve rapid, and often dramatic, results. Anyone who has used *Belladonna* for sunstroke, *Apis* for a bee-sting, or *Arnica* for a bruise or strain, can attest to the fact that merely a few pellets of the right medicine under the tongue can alleviate symptoms within minutes. It can be a bit more challenging to select the correct medicine for acute illnesses, and the results can take hours or even a few days, but they can be just as successful.

Success builds upon success. Once you discover that homeopathy can cure your bladder infection or motion sickness, you will feel much more willing to use it again the next time you have a first-aid or acute problem. The following guidelines will allow you to treat yourself quite effectively:

- Make sure your condition is either first-aid or acute, not chronic.
- Treat yourself as soon as possible after the problem first arises.
- Be sure to get emergency or professional help if appropriate.
- Feel free to supplement homeopathy with other interventions, as indicated for each condition.
- Carefully follow the instructions for self-prescribing the homeopathic medicines.

You will need to determine when you can help yourself and when you should seek help from a homeopath or other health-care provider. The first step in doing so is to identify what type of illness needs to be treated.

FIRST-AID CONDITIONS

These include urgent situations such as cuts and scrapes, sprains and strains, bruises, burns, insect bites and stings, sunstroke or heatstroke, and injuries. Homeopathy can be extraordinarily beneficial in these situations, sometimes in combination with emergency measures or, if necessary, transport to the emergency room of your local hospital. Selecting a homeopathic medicine for first-aid situations is generally very simple and straightforward. It is beyond the focus of this book, however, to discuss homeopathic first-aid medicines. Please consult *Homeopathic Self-Care: The Quick and Easy Guide for the Whole Family,* or a similar book, for first-aid guidelines.

MINOR ACUTE ILLNESSES

Acute illnesses by definition are of sudden onset, short duration, and self-limiting. This means literally that a woman suffering from an acute illness will either recover on her own over time or will die from this illness relatively quickly. Acute conditions can either be minor, such as the common cold, or severe, such as appendicitis. Minor acute illnesses include colds, coughs, the flu, sore throats, and diarrhea. Some minor acute women's complaints are bladder infections, mastitis, morning sickness, and vaginal infections. Acute emotional states include grief, anxiety, and fear of flying.

You will be pleasantly surprised by how easy it is to use homeopathy for such minor illnesses. When your self-prescribing is successful, you may be able to eliminate or cut down on visits to doctors and the emergency room.

SEVERE ACUTE ILLNESSES

Some acute illnesses, though short-lived, are quite severe. The pain can be intense and unrelenting and the complications serious or even life-threatening, such as with an ectopic pregnancy, gallbladder attack, or kidney stone. A knowledgeable and experienced homeopath may be able to treat even severe acute illnesses with considerable success, but these medical problems are clearly beyond the scope of this book. There is a big difference between what you can learn from applying the information in this book and from having ten to twenty years' experience as a professional homeopath. A little knowledge can be wonderfully empowering or a dangerous thing, so know and respect your limits.

The *perception* of the severity of an acute illness can be just as important as, or even more so than, the reality. Let me give you an interesting example.

Lydia's Story

Lydia, whom I have treated with homeopathy for nearly ten years, called my office not too long ago for advice about her bad cold. When she first spoke to our receptionist, she complained, "I can't stand this any longer and I'm about to go get antibiotics." This surprised me since she had always had great confidence in homeopathy.

When I spoke with Lydia an hour or so later, she lamented that she felt desperate. She considered her suffering unbearable and felt that she just couldn't go on any longer. Upon my inquiring further about the precise nature of her symptoms, it became clear that Lydia was not in any pain.

"What then," I explored, "is so unbearable?" Lydia explained that she had just lost her mom to cancer and had spent the previous month nursing her through her final days. She had missed so much work already and her co-workers had generously filled in during her absence. Now that she had completed her family duties, she needed to get back to her work responsibilities. Otherwise, she might as well die.

It's a good thing I knew Lydia well or her apparently disproportional despair over a chest cold would not have made sense. She again needed a homeopathic medicine that had helped her greatly during her infrequent times of serious depression in the past: *Aurum metallicum* (gold). Lydia was so deeply entrenched in her darkness that even though I assured her she would feel better by the next day, she was dubious. She had a friend pick up the *Aurum* at our office and left a message the next day assuring me that she felt much, much better. When I next saw her several weeks later, she reiterated that her cold and depression had both lifted almost immediately and had not returned.

This is an example of an acute illness with such a severe mental picture that it needed to be treated by a homeopath. Under normal circumstances, however, you might effectively treat your own chest cold with homeopathy, particularly if you treat it early on.

CHRONIC CONDITIONS

These include longstanding illnesses such as irritable bowel syndrome, colitis, eczema, asthma, headaches, depression, and eating disorders. Some common chronic women's conditions are menstrual problems, PMS, herpes, endometriosis, uterine fibroids, infertility, and osteoporosis. These problems, though they may respond quite well to homeopathic treatment under the care of an experienced professional, are not good candidates for self-care. Selecting the correct homeopathic medicine can be very complex, particularly in chronic illness. Don't even attempt to treat yourself for such conditions. With the support of an experienced homeopath, your chances of healing may be very good. I estimate a 70 percent success rate with many women's conditions if you stick with homeopathic treatment for at least a year.

GUIDELINES FOR WHEN TO SELF-TREAT AND WHEN NOT TO

• *How long have you suffered with the acute illness?* The sooner you can treat an acute illness with homeopathy, the more likely you will have a rapid response. If it has dragged on for days or weeks, it may be more difficult to cure.

• *Are you reasonably sure of the diagnosis?* If this is a condition, such as a flu or cold or bladder infection, that you have had before and clearly recognize the symptoms again, you can be fairly certain of the diagnosis. If, on the other hand, you have severe abdominal pain that could be either a stomach flu, food poisoning, appendicitis, or an ectopic pregnancy, get help, homeopathic or otherwise.

• *Is your acute condition serious?* Certain women's problems, such as a bladder infection, if left untreated or inappropriately treated, can sometimes quickly turn into something more severe, like a kidney infection. In the case of a miscarriage, you need to be certain there is no retained tissue, which can cause a serious, even life-threatening, infection. Nausea of pregnancy, if severe and persistent, can result in dehydration, requiring hospitalization and intravenous fluids. Know your limits and consult a qualified medical practitioner if you have any doubts or questions about treating yourself, and seek professional help if your symptoms persist.

• *Is your problem really acute?* Acute and chronic problems are handled very differently in homeopathy. The relatively simple procedure I describe for self-care for acute women's conditions is quite straightforward compared to consulting a professional homeopath who takes an hour or two to investigate and explore all aspects of your health and nature to find a single medicine for all of you.

Homeopaths make a distinction between a *true acute illness*—in other words, one that is an occasional, short-lived flare-up—as opposed to *an acute exacerbation of a chronic illness.* The latter is a condition such as herpes, which is a chronic problem with periodic outbreaks. It would be a mistake to consider herpes an acute illness, and you would be unlikely to have much success treating it with homeopathy unless your whole person was addressed. True acute illnesses, such as an infrequent episode of a bladder infection, can be treated quite effectively with self-care. If, however, the bladder infections become part of a recurrent pattern, it will be much more beneficial for you to consider them a chronic illness and consult a homeopath who can help you eliminate your underlying predisposition to get them in the first place.

- *Is this problem just one of many health problems?* If the acute women's problem that you wish to self-treat is an isolated concern and you are otherwise healthy, there is a good chance that you can find a medicine to help you. If, however, in addition to your hemorrhoids you have anxiety and irritable bowel syndrome, or in addition to your menstrual pain you have a history of irregular periods, PMS, and depression, you are not a good candidate for homeopathic self-care. Perhaps you might be able to help yourself with your cramps, but the extent to which you could be helped by constitutional homeopathy is so much greater that you would be shortsighted to limit your potential healing.

- *Are you under the care of a homeopath?* If so, check with her regarding her preference about your treating yourself for an acute condition. Attitudes vary from one practitioner to another.

- *Is a significant mental or emotional state associated with the acute illness?* If the acute illness is accompanied by severe fright or despair (such as with Lydia), let a homeopath treat you. The results will be much better, and your mental state as well as the physical problem will be addressed.

- *Are you taking conventional medications for the acute condition?* This is a bit more complicated and probably requires professional help, although, if the medications are over-the-counter, self-treatment is generally fine.

- *How long have you been trying to treat the condition homeopathically without a significant improvement?* If your acute condition is mild and homeopathic self-prescribing hasn't helped you within a week, get help. If your situation is of moderate severity, give yourself a couple of days unless your symptoms take a turn for the worse. In more serious conditions, you may have time to try one medicine, if it closely matches your symptoms, otherwise, seek immediate help.

PART TWO

Healing Yourself with Homeopathy for Acute Women's Problems

Taking an Acute Homeopathic Case

Knowing How to Ask the Right Questions

WHEN TO USE THIS SECTION TO TREAT YOURSELF

This part of the book is designed to help you find the best medicine to help you self-treat more minor or acute problems. If you have any doubt as to whether your problem falls into this category, please reread chapter 6, which defines and explains the different kinds of illnesses, what can be self-treated, and what cannot. Remember that if you need help with any longstanding or persistent problem, one that recurs on a regular basis, or one that is severe, it is best to consult a professional homeopath. Those types of problems are well beyond the scope of what is described in this chapter. They require much more extensive and complicated casetaking, and expertise and case management that can only be developed after years of homeopathic practice. You won't do yourself any favors in such situations, by trying to act as your own doctor, and you may prolong your suffering by delaying effective treatment.

If you use this section of the book to treat the appropriate type of condition, by following my guidelines, you will quite likely be pleased with the results. Homeopathy can work very quickly, and often dramatically, in acute illnesses, especially if the treatment begins as early as possible. If no homeopathic medicine is clearly indicated, or if you wish to add other therapies as well, I have included a number of other tried-and-true recommendations that I have used with women over the past sixteen years.

MASTERING AN ART

If you like putting together jigsaw puzzles, you'll love homeopathic casetaking! What you will do is assemble the pieces of your symptom picture, one by one, until the puzzle is complete. Once the pieces are all in the right place and the image is identifiable, you can match it to a medicine to produce an excellent result. If any of the key pieces is missing, the image may not be clear enough to find the right medicine. Carefully ask yourself all of the indicated questions, make all the recommended observations, and patiently think about everything that contributed to your acute illness. Don't rush through this stage, because each and every symptom is potentially quite important. The better you take your own case, the more quickly your suffering will likely pass.

USING THE LOOK, LISTEN, AND ASK SECTIONS

The first step in treating yourself is identifying the problem. Select the women's condition that you think best fits your own, such as a bladder infection, mastitis, or morning sickness. Double-check to make sure that the description of the problem and symptoms matches yours and take a look at the possible complications to make sure it is safe to treat yourself without the help of an expert. If you find that your symptoms do not fit the diagnosis you suspected, you need to change course and select the appropriate diagnosis. If your diagnosis remains confusing, complicated, or unclear, either find a professional homeopath who can treat you or seek other medical assistance.

The Look, Listen, and Ask sections that appear under each condition are designed to carefully guide you through your self-casetaking process so that you can gather all of the information necessary to choose the best medicine. The Look section (designated by the eye icon) teaches you what to observe, the Listen section (ear icon) details what you are most likely to hear yourself say about what's going on (either to others or to yourself), and the Ask section (question mark icon) offers specific questions to ask yourself about your problem.

Look

The first thing to do in order to understand what is happening with yourself and to treat yourself homeopathically is to observe. When you feel sick, a number of things may change: the color and expression of your face; your posture, energy, state of mind, and mood; what you feel like eating, drinking, or doing; or whether you want anyone else to be around. What changes when you become acutely ill is very important in terms of finding a homeopathic medicine to help you.

Looking takes into account everything that you can observe about yourself. Allow yourself to use each of your five senses, as well as your sixth, intuition. Notice whether you usually have a sunny disposition and are now a growly bear, or whether you are normally the eager beaver yet now are a lump, draped over your favorite couch. Do you guzzle water much more than usual? Do you generally prefer a brisk breeze but now find yourself huddling by the heater, shivering? All of these shifts are an important part of your homeopathic picture—a piece of the puzzle you will put together in order to *solve your case,* as homeopathic Sherlock Holmes–types are prone to say.

Take a survey of yourself and be sure to include anything and everything that has changed since you developed your acute problem. I will guide you as to what specific features are of particular importance in each individual condition.

Listen

Participate in a dialogue with yourself—a self-interview. You can do it aloud or silently, whichever way is easiest for you to check in with yourself. Start with open-ended questions like, "How do I feel? What's going on? What happened just before this problem came on? Which specific symptoms most bother me and what makes them better or worse?" Notice what you feel as you answer these questions. Is a particular mood or state of mind associated with your symptoms?

Ask

Although I think that just about anything that has changed since your particular problem developed is relevant, having taken women's acute cases for years, I find certain questions to be consistently useful. I include this list along with each women's condition. It's kind of like having me or another experienced homeopath right beside you, whispering in your ear so that you can best know which questions to ask yourself.

There are three types of symptoms in taking a homeopathic case: *mental and emotional, physical general,* and *physical particular.* Mental and emotional symptoms include thoughts, feelings, perceptions, dreams, fears, and all other psychological features. Physical general symptoms are those you experience throughout your body, such as sleepiness, hunger, a fever, or perspiration. Physical particular symptoms are physical symptoms pertaining to an individual part of your body, such as an itching sensation in the labia, cramping in the right ovary, or burning in the urethra. You will find both general and particular symptoms listed under each medicine in the Women's Conditions and *Materia Medica* chapters of the book.

Another important clue to sorting out your symptoms is a *modality.* A modality is what makes an individual symptom better or worse and is another way in which your symptom is unique. Taking the symptoms I just mentioned, a modality would be labial itching that was worse after taking a warm bath, right ovarian pain that felt better from lying on the right side of your body, or burning in the urethra that you experienced just as you finished urinating. Modalities are only important if they significantly alter the symptom, not if they make only a minor and temporary difference.

STRANGE, RARE, AND PECULIAR

When I take an acute case, one factor is singly the most important in selecting a homeopathic medicine. This is what stands out as most unusual in the case, something that is quite different from what I normally hear women tell me. Homeopaths call such a symptom *strange, rare, and peculiar*. It is out of the ordinary, unexpected. For instance, many people with asthma or other obstructive lung conditions breathe more easily when they are propped up in bed. This is common. But if your asthma is relieved by lying perfectly flat in bed or with your head lower than your torso, it is a strange, rare, and peculiar symptom. Similarly, breast swelling before the menstrual period is a common complaint of many women. If your breasts became enlarged and tender *after* your period, this is more unusual, of greater interest to a homeopath, and considerably more useful in helping you or your homeopath select a medicine.

YOUR STATE

Equally important, if not more important than the specific physical symptoms, is your *state*. This includes your attitude, temperament, and nature. Your interests, dress, relationship preferences, livelihood, health—in fact, everything about you—are a reflection of your state. Many homeopaths place considerable emphasis on your state in selecting a constitutional medicine. It can also be helpful in acute prescribing and is reflected by the mental and emotional symptoms that accompany the problem or that have changed since the onset of the problem, as well as by any psychological factors that brought about the acute illness in the first place.

You might think that you just happened to get a cold because your partner or colleague sneezed on you. Or that you got a vaginal yeast infection because you took antibiotics—that an acute illness is something you catch in a rather random and haphazard fashion. A homeopath, on the other hand, views acute illnesses as part of the overall package of your predispositions, vulnerability, vitality, and state. Yes, upper respiratory infections can be viral and antibiotics do indiscriminately kill off the good vaginal flora as well as the bad. But not every one of your colleagues will catch that cold and not every woman who takes antibiotics will subsequently develop vaginal yeast. Above all, whether or not you become acutely ill depends on the strength of your vital force, hereditary predisposition, and your physical, mental, and emotional state at the time of the exposure. If they are all in balance, no matter how virulent the virus or how strong the antibiotic, you will stay healthy.

A SAMPLE SELF-CASETAKING

Q: What you ask yourself
A: Your reply

Q: What's the problem?
A: I think I have a bladder infection.

Q: What makes you think that?
A: I have to urinate a lot and it hurts.

Q: When did this start?
A: This morning when I woke up.

Q: What happened right before you got the bladder infection?
A: I made love with my new boyfriend, Jim, for the first time. We've been dating for months but this is the first time we actually had sexual intercourse. We're really attracted to each other and I think we got a bit carried away. I forgot to get up and urinate afterward. This morning I woke up to go to the bathroom and it hurt. And I have to go to the bathroom every fifteen minutes.

Q: What's the pain like?
A: It burns where the urine comes out after I finish going to the bathroom.

Q: Any other symptoms?
A: No, just the pain and having to urinate more often.

Q: How did you feel yesterday before you made love?
A: Actually, we got into a bit of a fight because he told me I'm overly sensitive and can't handle criticism. It really hurt my feelings. Then we made up and had a wonderful night.

Q: Anything else?
A: No.

Q: Have you ever had a bladder infection before?
A: Once before, about ten years ago, right after I made love with my very first boyfriend. It was actually quite similar. I ended up taking antibiotics. It's funny. This issue of getting my feelings hurt used to come up a lot with him, too.

Q: Does anything make the pain or urinary frequency better or worse?
A: If I keep drinking a lot of water, the pain's not so bad, but I have the urge to go to the bathroom even more.

If you hadn't stopped to think about your symptoms in depth and had immediately gone to your doctor for antibiotics, you might never have made the connection between your hurt feelings and the bladder infection. Your doctor would have probably found out that you had made love the night before but not delved any more deeply into your emotions because she would have given you the same antibiotic, regardless. Even by going through this process yourself, you can gain a lot more insight into your patterns and tendencies and become empowered to change in a very deep way.

There are two thousand or so possible medicines in homeopathy, not just a handful of antibiotics. In this case, if these were your symptoms, *Staphysagria* would likely not only bring about rapid relief of your urethral discomfort but, if prescribed on a constitutional level, would probably help you to become stronger and less vulnerable to hurt feelings, as well as prevent future bladder infections.

RECORDING YOUR CASE FOR THE FUTURE

Write down all of your symptoms, the medicines that you considered and why, the potency of the chosen medicine, the frequency with which you took it, and the results. This is helpful for a number of reasons:

- If you treat the condition successfully and then experience the symptoms again one or several years later, you can look back at what worked and save the time, trouble, and suffering of choosing one or more incorrect medicines or giving a potency that is not exactly right.
- If the condition does *not* respond to your treatment, you can take your notes to a homeopath so that she can see what you already took and for what reasons, as well as see the progression of the acute illness.
- If you decide to study homeopathy more seriously, having a record of your self-care can be quite instructive.

One way to make your casetaking more clear is to indicate in some way the most important symptoms in your case. Here are three ways to do this:

1. <u>Underline</u> once the symptoms that are somewhat clear, mildly intense, and come out upon questioning. <u>Underline twice</u> those symptoms that are clearer, more intense, and come up immediately or spontaneously. <u>Underline three times</u> the symptoms that are extremely clear, quite intense, and seem to be the most important.

2. Instead of underlining, give the equivalent of a once-underlined symptom a (1), a twice-underlined symptom a (2), and use (3) for three underlines.

3. Circle any symptoms that are especially significant.

The purpose of these techniques is to help you visually differentiate the most important from the least important symptoms so that you can do a self-analysis of your case, choose a medicine quickly, and be able to look back at your case easily at a later date.

Keep all of your case records in a notebook filed by year so that you can consult them later or show them to your homeopath. I find it very helpful in my patient charts to keep a list on the top of the left-hand side of the chart, easily visible, with the date the medicine was prescribed, type of problem, name of the medicine, potency, and result. This will make prescribing years later for the same symptoms a breeze, without my having to sift through pages of previous self-prescriptions.

CHAPTER 8

Choosing the Best Homeopathic Medicine

The Closer the Match, the Better the Result

ANALYZING YOUR CASE

Once you have gathered the necessary information from your casetaking, you are ready to put it all together in order to select the one medicine that will most likely bring you rapid relief. If you follow these steps, the process will be relatively straight-forward, depending on how well you take your own case and how clearly your symptoms match a homeopathic medicine.

   1. **Read the Description of the Appropriate Women's Condition**   I have included the conditions in chapter 11 that are most suitable for self-treatment. If your condition is there, proceed. If not, it is likely to be beyond the scope of your treating yourself. Consult chapter 13 and, if your problem appears there, read the corresponding section, then find a qualified and experienced homeopathic practitioner. If you have an acute condition that is not a women's condition, per se, you will probably find it covered in my general book *Homeopathic Self-Care: The Quick and Easy Guide for the Whole Family,* which includes the seventy most common acute problems.

Assuming that your condition is included in chapter 11, read the description of the problem and the symptoms to make sure you have diagnosed yourself correctly. It is not uncommon, for example, to confuse a bladder infection with vaginitis, so make sure the diagnosis fits because the medicines and recommendations are entirely different. It's a good idea to take a look at the Complications section just to make sure you can't get into any trouble by not seeing a health-care practitioner.

2. Read the Pointers and the Listen Sections   The Pointers for Finding Your Homeopathic Medicine give brief summaries of the most commonly used homeopathic medicines for each women's problem, along with the features that distinguish them most readily. The Listen section contains expressive phrases similar to those I hear my patients say when they need each particular medicine.

3. Read the Description of Each Indicated Homeopathic Medicine

- Read the Key Symptoms.
- If you have mental and emotional symptoms, read the Mind section. If your case is purely physical or if none of the mental symptoms listed match your own, disregard them.
- Read the Body section.
- Read the Worse and Better sections.
- Read the Food and Drink section if your preferences or aversions have changed since the problem began or are quite marked.

I have described each homeopathic medicine based on the most characteristic pattern of symptoms for which it is likely to be effective with a particular problem. As you read about each medicine, ask yourself how closely it fits your own symptoms. You may not have *all* of the symptoms that are listed for the medicine you consider, but the symptoms you *do* have should mostly fit. The descriptions, though brief, cover the most commonly presenting symptoms of each medicine. Read *across* the chart to find all of the symptoms for the medicine of choice and *down* the chart to compare the features of the different medicines.

SELECTING THE BEST MEDICINE FOR YOU

You are trying to find the best possible match among the medicines listed. I have included those that you will most likely need, as well as, in certain conditions, some less commonly prescribed medicines. Realize that there are over two thousand homeopathic medicines. If your symptoms do *not* clearly match those of the medicines listed, it doesn't mean that homeopathy cannot help you, but rather that your presenting picture is not one of the most commonplace ones and is likely to need a more unusual medicine and an experienced homeopath to find it. If several medicines have some characteristics that are in your own case, read each one in the *Materia Medica* section, which lists fifty common medicines I use for acute women's conditions and their main indications and characteristics.

There are two ways to use this section of the book to find the best homeopathic medicine to treat yourself:

1. Read the corresponding symptoms for each medicine listed under your condition. From this, you will get a good idea of what a woman with *your* problem needing *that* medicine will be like.

2. Read the *Materia Medica* in chapter 14 for any medicine that you consider, to gain a more in-depth understanding of its indications for a variety of different problems. You will get a better idea of whether or not it matches your case and, since each medicine treats many symptoms and conditions, a taste of the wide range of possibilities for each medicine in helping women.

Now that you are more informed about the pool of medicines from which to choose, discard those that do not fit your symptoms. Select the one that is the closest match, although perhaps not a perfect one. No woman can present with *all* of the symptoms of a given medicine. You are searching for the medicine whose symptom picture is *most* similar to your own.

To make the process even easier, you may want to divide your symptoms into Key Symptoms, Mind, Body, Worse, and Better so that you can more readily recognize your symptom pattern and match it to the description of a given medicine. The **bold-faced** symptoms listed under each medicine are the ones that I have seen most often in women patients presenting with that complaint, needing that medicine. If you have symptoms that you have underlined two or three times—in other words, that are quite intense and clear—it is probable that the symptom will be in boldface under the description of the medicine.

Choose the one medicine that is the best match. If no medicine matches well and you are sure you have all the information needed to make a differentiation, use the naturopathic recommendations for that condition, wait until your symptoms are clearer, or consult a homeopath.

CHAPTER 9

Once You Have Selected a Medicine

How, When, and How Often to Take It

ONE MEDICINE UNDER YOUR TONGUE

Homeopathic medicines come in the form of small-to-tiny white globules, pellets, or pills. They are meant to be taken orally. Although a small number of homeopaths administer the medicines in a water preparation, the more common procedure is to place them in the mouth under the tongue and allow them to dissolve. Since the medicines are infused in sugar pellets, even babies find them tasty and often want more. Once you have decided on your medicine of choice, take it, follow my guidelines for how to assess your improvement, and do not combine it with another medicine. It is best to:

- Avoid touching the pellets. Use a clean piece of paper or spoon to place them under the tongue without touching them.
- Wait at least five minutes before eating or drinking.
- If you are chewing gum or have just brushed your teeth, wait ten minutes until the odor and taste are gone before taking the pill.
- Don't take other medicines at the very same time.

POSSIBLE SCENARIOS ONCE YOU HAVE TAKEN A MEDICINE

After you have taken a homeopathic medicine, one of the situations on the following pages will unfold.

No Change

What is happening   You are neither better nor worse. Your symptoms remain the same.

What to do   If you have taken three doses of the chosen medicine over a twenty-four-hour period with no improvement, you have not selected the correct medicine. If the problem is very acute and painful, such as a bladder infection, you should notice a definite improvement within an hour. If the problem has bothered you for a number of weeks, even a slight improvement merits waiting another day to monitor the progression of your illness. If the acute problem is of more recent onset or severe, you are likely to notice a significant positive response, usually within twelve hours after taking the medicine. If this does not occur, find another medicine and take it. If no medicine seems to fit, wait until your symptoms shift, try instead the other naturopathic recommendations I have included, or find an experienced homeopath to help you.

> Example:
> *You take* Cantharis *for a urinary infection but are no better within an hour. You restudy your case, switch to* Staphysagria, *and feel better within fifteen minutes.*

A Clear but Partial Improvement

What is happening   Your symptoms are less intense. Some have gone away entirely. You feel perkier and more yourself. The medicine has begun to act in a positive way.

What to do   Wait for further improvement. Do not take another dose unless you start to feel worse again in the same way as before.

> Example:
> *You take* Sepia *for morning sickness. You notice that your nausea is 30 percent better after three days, but, knowing that morning sickness is one of the conditions for which it is best to wait a week to ten days before changing to another medicine, you give it more time. After eight days, all of your symptoms are 90 percent better.*

Complete, Rapid Relief

What is happening   All of your symptoms go away quickly. You feel great.

What to do   Be happy that you picked just the right medicine for you.

Example:

You're out on a whale-watch boat and the water is getting rough. You start to feel awful. Being wisely prepared, you brought this book and a medicine kit with you. Tabacum *sounds like a perfect match. You take it and within ten minutes you feel like a new woman. Aren't those humpbacks outrageous?*

Your Symptoms Become Worse and Do Not Get Better

What is happening   You took the medicine twelve hours ago and feel no better. Some of your symptoms are worse, but basically you feel just like you did before you took the medicine.

What to do   It is most likely that there is a better medicine for you. Did you do anything that might have interfered with the medicine (see pages 175–176 for antidoting substances)? If you have an acute flare-up of a chronic condition, you may not have waited long enough to evaluate it. Assuming these are not the case, look for another medicine that matches your symptoms more closely. Remember to emphasize what is most striking or unusual about your symptoms. If you find a better medicine, take it. If you have been exposed to an antidoting factor, stop using it and take the first medicine again. Otherwise, use the naturopathic recommendations for your problem and/or seek professional homeopathic help or other medical care.

Example:

You took Belladonna *for your mastitis. Even after forty-eight hours your breasts were terribly sore and tender. You reread the list of antidoting substances and realized you were using Chapstick at the same time. You toss the lip balm, repeat the* Belladonna, *and within twenty-four hours your breast pain is 75 percent improved.*

Your Symptoms Become Worse, Then You Get Much Better

What is happening   You feel worse for four hours, then considerably better.

What to do   You've chosen the right medicine. Wait. Repeat the medicine only if the same symptoms return.

Example:

You chose Hamamelis *for your hemorrhoids. Within fifteen minutes your hemorrhoid pain is much worse and lasts for another twenty minutes. Then it subsides over the next hour and does not return.*

Your Original Symptoms Change or Go Away and You Develop New Ones

What is happening   Your symptom picture is changing.

What to do   Restudy your case to see if there is a better medicine. If so, take it. Continue to monitor your symptoms. If the homeopathic medicines do not help and your symptoms progress rapidly or become severe, seek professional or emergency medical care. Your initial self-diagnosis may have been incorrect.

> Example:
> *You suspect gallbladder pain and take a dose of* Chelidonium. *Within an hour the pain is much more severe and your entire abdomen is ultrasensitive. You feel quite nauseous. Your partner takes you to the emergency room and you are diagnosed with appendicitis.*

WHEN TO REPEAT A HOMEOPATHIC MEDICINE

Less is better with homeopathy. You only need to repeat a medicine when it has worked and the effects wear off.

The Most Common Situation

You may either:

1. Take the medicine one time only. Once you clearly improve, repeat it only if you start to feel worse again.
2. If you are taking the medicine on a schedule, such as every two to four hours until you notice an improvement, repeat if you relapse. Stop when you see an improvement.

Other Guidelines

• If your symptoms are severe and of rapid onset, such as an extremely painful mastitis or bladder infection, you may need to take doses more frequently.

• In case of an emergency or very severe problem, such as an excruciatingly painful miscarriage, you may need to repeat the medicine as often as every fifteen to thirty minutes, in addition to seeking appropriate medical attention.

• If your symptoms develop slowly and are of mild to moderate severity, you will not have to repeat the medicine as often.

Repeat the Medicine

1. Up to three times, every two to four hours, depending on the potency, until you start to feel better.
2. When your symptoms return after you felt better, even if the improvement was brief.
3. When your original symptoms return.
4. If the medicine has been antidoted.

• If you develop an aggravation (your symptoms become worse) after taking a dose of a medicine, do not take another dose until the aggravation has subsided and only at that time if you improved, then relapsed.

• If you have taken three doses of a medicine without any improvement, take the next best medicine as long as you have eliminated the possibility of an antidoting influence.

• If you are confused about what to do, wait and do nothing. Observe yourself and it will become clear what to do next.

CHANGING THE MEDICINE

You should feel significantly better, generally at least 50 to 90 percent, after taking the correct homeopathic medicine. If the first one does not clearly help, choose a second. A medicine that is similar to the correct one may have a partial, but not a dramatic or lasting, effect.

You Slowly Improve

What is happening   You improve gradually but steadily.

What to do   Don't change the medicine, even if the improvement seems slow. Some women's conditions take longer than others to respond to homeopathy and, as long as you are definitely improving, the likelihood is high that you have chosen the right medicine.

> Example:
> *You took* Sepia *because you felt blue after your baby was born. Ten days later you feel 30 percent better and your energy is starting to pick up again. You wait another ten days and notice that you feel 75 percent better.*

Your Symptom Picture Shifts

What is happening   The first medicine you took acted, but then your symptoms shifted. The first medicine may have been close but not completely correct.

What to do   Base your choice of medicines on what is happening at the moment. If the symptoms have changed to any significant degree in an acute illness, you most likely need a new medicine.

> Example:
> *You took* Staphysagria *for a bladder infection. The bladder discomfort improved, but now the pain has moved down to the urethra and matches the picture of* Sarsaparilla. *You take it and your urinary infection goes away completely.*

Change the Medicine

1. If the first medicine has no effect. As long as the first medicine helps you, even if the improvement is gradual, do not change the medicine.
2. If the symptoms change markedly, change the medicine. Repeat it only as needed.
3. If the original medicine helped but no longer works.

CHAPTER **10**

Your Women's Homeopathic Self-Care Medicine Kit

Make Sure You Have the Medicines You Need

HAVE YOUR KIT WITH YOU WHEN YOU NEED IT!

One of the great advantages of homeopathy is the negligible expense of the medicines. A month's supply of many conventional medicines can cost fifty to one hundred dollars or more. This amount of money could easily buy a year's worth of homeopathic medicines. They are inexpensive and, in the case of constitutional treatment under the care of a homeopath, one medicine treats all of you so you don't need to keep a list of a dozen or more different medicines or vitamins to remember what you're taking. In addition to these advantages, homeopathic medicines have no expiration date and only need to be replaced when the bottle is empty.

You can learn a lot from this book about helping yourself for acute women's problems, but you won't get very far with homeopathy unless you have the medicines you need. The best time to take a medicine is right after the onset of the problem, so the handier the medicines are, the better. No matter where I go, I try to take along a traveling homeopathic kit. One exception, unfortunately, was during a homeopathic conference in Hawaii where, on a snorkeling cruise to the island of Molokini off Maui, I became hopelessly seasick. I was thoroughly miserable and surrounded by a boatload of other homeopaths; not a single one of us had our medicine kits with us. I learned my lesson that day!

I have put together a self-care kit that goes along with this book. It is the only kit that I know of containing the fifty medicines I find most useful for women who wish to treat themselves. An order form is included in the back of the book. A variety of other kits containing acute medicines for general conditions, such as my *Homeopathic Self-Care Home Medicine Kit,* are available. A number of the medicines included in this book will not be sold at your local health food store. All of the medicines mentioned in this book are *single* homeopathic medicines, as opposed to *combination* medicines containing several or many different homeopathic medicines.

Regardless of which kit you buy, have it when and where you need it. At home, at school, at work, in your car, on your travels—wherever you are most likely to have problems. As you can see from the example of my Molokini experience, there is nothing more frustrating than knowing just which homeopathic medicine *you* need (I desperately needed *Tabacum*) and not being able to get it!

WHAT TO INCLUDE IN YOUR KIT

I recommend using a kit that contains 30C potency medicines. Some kits contain 6X, 12X, 12C, or 30X potencies. While a well-chosen homeopathic medicine should work in any potency, the disadvantage of these lower-potency kits is that a dose needs to be repeated quite often, sometimes up to six times a day. It is much easier to use a 30C potency, which can be taken up to every four hours at the most, and often only two or three times in all. In my practice, I tend to use much higher potencies, such as 200C, 1M, and 10M, but I do not suggest your using them without extensive knowledge of and experience with homeopathy.

I include the following medicines in the Women's Self-Care Medicine Kit:

Aconite	*Cimicifuga*
Aesculus	*Cocculus*
Apis	*Coffea*
Arnica	*Colchicum*
Arsenicum	*Collinsonia*
Belladonna	*Colocynthis*
Bellis perennis	*Conium*
Bryonia	*Folliculinum*
Cactus	*Gelsemium*
Caladium	*Hamamelis*
Calcarea carbonica	*Ignatia*
Cantharis	*Kreosotum*
Castor equi	*Lac caninum*
Caulophyllum	*Lachesis*
Chamomilla	*Lactuca*
China	*Lycopodium*

Magnesium phosphorica
Mercurius corrosivus
Natrum muriaticum
Nux vomica
Petroleum
Phellandrium
Phosphorus
Phytolacca
Pulsatilla

Sabina
Sanguinaria
Sarsaparilla
Sepia
Silica
Staphysagria
Sulphur
Tabacum
Veratrum album

HOW TO TAKE CARE OF YOUR MEDICINES

Homeopathic medicines can last a lifetime (unless they run out, of course) as long as you follow a few precautions:

- Avoid touching the pellets with your hands.
- Open one bottle at a time so you won't be confused about which medicine is which or contaminate the bottles.
- If a medicine spills, throw it away.
- Store your kit away from direct sunlight, extreme heat, and aromatic substances that act as possible antidotes (see pages 175–176).
- When traveling, just to be on the safe side, pass your kit around the airport x-ray machines.

CHAPTER **11**

Conditions You Can Self-Treat Safely and Effectively

NAVIGATING THE ICONS

This section can be used in a number of ways: to confirm your suspected acute diagnosis, to learn about potential complications, to find a homeopathic medicine that can help you, and to know how often to take it and what to expect. It also offers practical naturopathic recommendations that can be very beneficial, either alone or in combination with homeopathy.

Choose the Appropriate Condition

1. Select the condition that most closely resembles your own.
2. Read the description and symptoms to make sure you're on the right path.

Read About the Condition

 Description
Defines the condition and what causes it.

 Symptoms
Describes the common symptoms of the condition.

Complications

Tells you about potential problems, medical emergencies, and when you need medical assistance.

Use the Look, Listen, and Ask Sections to Help You Take Your Case

Look

Offers you tips on what to observe about yourself.

Listen

Guides you in your inner dialogue about what's going on with you, relative to the characteristic symptoms of indicated homeopathic medicines.

Ask

Provides you with specific questions to find out more about your symptoms.

Read the Pointers Section for Finding the Homeopathic Medicine

Pointers for Finding Your Homeopathic Medicine

Gives you brief summaries of typical symptoms and indicates which medicines should be considered for those types of symptoms.

Use the Chart of the Homeopathic Medicines

You may choose to read the chart either vertically or horizontally:

- If you read *down* the column of Key Symptoms, you can compare the medicines for a particular type of symptoms.
- If you read *across,* you will learn the range of symptoms for a particular medicine.

1. First read Key Symptoms for especially strong or striking symptoms that are characteristic of the particular homeopathic medicine.

2. Read the Mind section next for important mental and emotional symptoms characteristic of the medicine.

3. Read the Body portion next to learn about other physical symptoms covered by the medicine.

4. Read the Worse section for the factors that can adversely affect you if this is the medicine that matches your symptom picture.

5. Read the Better section for the factors that can affect you positively if this is the medicine that matches your symptom picture.

6. Read the Food and Drink section to get an idea of which foods and beverages you will likely want or reject and how hungry or thirsty you might be if you need the particular medicine.

Compare Symptoms

Compare the symptoms you have gathered about your problem with those listed for each medicine.

- Pay special attention to the Key Symptoms.
- If you have no mental symptoms with the acute illness, skip past the Mind section, but if you do have new or unusual mental symptoms, be sure to take them into account.
- Take special notice of the other Body symptoms listed and compare them to your own.
- Match the factors that aggravate or alleviate your symptoms with those in the Worse and Better categories.
- If you have any strong desires for food or drinks or are significantly more or less hungry or thirsty than normal, compare those with the ones listed under Food and Drink.

Read About the Medicines

Flip to *Materia Medica* (chapter 14) and read about the medicines you might consider.

- Check to see whether any of your *other* symptoms are listed for the medicine(s).
- Double-check to see if there is a good match between your symptoms and the overall impression you receive from reading about the medicine.

Choose the Best Medicine

Most, but rarely all, of your symptoms should be covered by the medicine you choose. You may also have *other* symptoms that are not listed. That is fine. I could have listed pages of symptoms for each medicine if space allowed. The medicine that appears to match most closely is probably the correct one for you.

After Selecting a Medicine

Dosage
Read this part to find out how to take the medicine.

What to Expect from Homeopathic Women's Self-Care
Read this section to give yourself a realistic time frame for getting better.

Naturopathic Recommendations for Women's Self-Care
These are other natural and practical tips I would give you if I were there to help and support you.

WHAT YOU CAN EXPECT WITH HOMEOPATHIC SELF-CARE

You will likely have excellent results if you carefully follow the guidelines in this book. Remember to read the section in chapter 12 about substances and influences that can interfere with homeopathy. It is just as important to avoid them if you treat yourself as it is if you are treated by a professional homeopath. When practiced appropriately, homeopathy works! For many acute problems, you do not have to be an expert to get great results. Here is a wonderful example that I received by e-mail from Slovenia.

Katrina's Story

"I suffered from a bladder infection on my holiday abroad. When I returned to Slovenia, a laboratory test confirmed the diagnosis, but I refused to undergo the antibiotic treatment prescribed by both my urologist and my homeopath, who treats in both the homeopathic and the modern ways. I happened to buy your book *Homeopathic Self-Care* in a huge bookshop far away from my country. How I chose it among the mass of homeopathic literature, I can't tell you, but it looked systematic and practical.

"Looking through your book at the medicines for bladder infections, I immediately identified *Staphysagria* as the proper one for me. When I called my homeopath to ask him to send me that medicine, he assured me that I had chosen the right one and seemed surprised that I knew what I needed. Once I took the *Staphysagria*, my condition improved considerably, as confirmed by another urine test.

"Because of my first successful self-treatment, my confidence has risen. I hope that your extremely practical guide will soon be translated into Slovene."

Bladder Infection *(Acute, not Recurrent)*

Description

Bladder infections, caused by microorganisms that colonize the bladder, are fifty times more prevalent in women between the ages of twenty and fifty. You may have no apparent symptoms even though your bacterial culture is positive or you may experience symptoms without any evidence of infection.

Symptoms

If you have a bladder infection (cystitis), you will most likely experience an urgent desire to urinate; frequent urination; pain in the urethra (where the urine comes out) or bladder before, during, or after urination; and lower back pain. There may also be blood in your urine. Women commonly suffer from bladder infections after sex with a new partner, after having postponed urination, after becoming dehydrated, or following catheterization.

Bladder infections vary in intensity and onset, from excruciating and sudden pain to milder and more tolerable discomfort of more gradual onset.

Complications

Your biggest risk is of the bladder infection ascending up your ureter (the tube going from the bladder to the kidney) resulting in acute pyelonephritis, a serious infection of the kidneys. Urinary frequency and urgency, accompanied by pain along the sides of the mid-back and fever can indicate pyelonephritis, in which case you need immediate medical attention.

Look

Do you need to urinate frequently?

Do you have to hurry to the bathroom to make it in time?

Has the color of your urine changed?

Is there blood or sediment in your urine?

Do you need to urinate in an unusual position?

Listen

"I have a very swollen, stinging feeling in my urethra and bladder." *Apis mellifica*

"It burns terribly in my bladder when I go to the bathroom, my urine is bloody, and I can't seem to sit still. And it came on so fast!" *Cantharis*

"The urgency is extreme. I want to hold it back because it burns so badly when I urinate, but I can't." *Mercurius corrosivus*

"My urethra (where the urine comes out) burns most just as I finish urinating." *Sarsaparilla*

"It's so aggravating. I seem to get a bladder infection whenever I make love with a new partner." *Staphysagria*

Ask

When did my symptoms start? Was there a clear cause?

Did something happen emotionally right before my symptoms began?

How quickly did my symptoms come on?

How severe are my symptoms?

Am I in pain? Where? What type of pain do I feel?

Exactly when do I feel the pain?

What makes the pain better or worse?

Do I have to urinate more frequently than usual?

Do I have to run to the bathroom?

Am I noticing any back pain?

Pointers for Finding Your Homeopathic Medicine

• Consider *Apis mellifica* if your pain is primarily burning or stinging, the area is swollen, the last drops of urine feel scalding, and the urine will not come out easily.

• Take *Cantharis* if your pain is excruciating or your urine is bloody. *Cantharis* has the most extreme and sudden bladder symptoms.

• The three most common medicines for bladder infections in women are *Cantharis, Staphysagria,* and *Sarsaparilla.*

• If the most prominent symptom is frequent, intense urging with severe pain, take *Mercurius corrosivus*.

• If you have burning in your urethra as you finish urinating, the first medicine to think of is *Sarsaparilla*. If it doesn't work, take a look at *Staphysagria* or *Cantharis*.

• If your bladder infection came on after making love, consider *Staphysagria* as your first medicine of choice.

Dosage

• Take three pellets of 30C every one to two hours until you see an improvement.

• If you are no better after three doses, change medicines.

• After you first notice you have improved, take another dose only if your symptoms begin to return.

• Lower potencies (6X, 6C, and 30X) may need to be taken more often (every one to two hours, depending on the severity of the symptoms.

• Higher potencies (200X, 200C, and 1M) usually need to be taken only once but may need a repetition if the symptoms are severe or return after initial improvement.

What to Expect from Women's Homeopathic Self-Care

You will most likely experience rapid and significant relief if you start treating your bladder infection immediately, because symptoms can progress quite rapidly in some women.

Homeopathy can alleviate your pain and stimulate your immune system to eliminate the infectious microorganisms. Where inflammation is present without infection, homeopathic medicines are also effective. Acute homeopathic treatment will only address your immediate infection. Constitutional homeopathy is highly effective in reducing or eliminating the tendency to develop bladder infections (see page 190).

Naturopathic Recommendations for Women's Self-Care

• Drink as much water as you possibly can.

• Take cranberry concentrate or capsules every one to two hours to acidify your urine. Cranberry juice is adequate if that is all you have available, but the sugar content is high.

• Go to the bathroom as soon as you feel the urge. Do *not* put it off until you have time.

- During an infection, avoid horseback riding or other activities that put pressure on your urethra and bladder.
- Take bladder herbs such as Oregon grape, *Bucchu, Pipsissewa, Uva ursi*, and cornsilk every two hours until your symptoms improve. The dosage will depend on whether you take it in the form of a tea, capsules, or a tincture.
- If you tend to develop a bladder infection from getting chilled, bundle up and stay warm.
- Some women find that citrus fruits aggravate their cystitis. If so, avoid them.
- To avoid future infections, drink lots of water, urinate after sex, and as soon as you feel the urge.

	Key Symptoms	Mind	Body	Worse	Better	Food & Drink
Apis *(Honeybee)*	**Scalding urine, especially the last drops** / **Stinging, burning pains** / **Swelling of parts of the body**	**Busy** / **Active** / Irritable if crossed	Urination is frequent and can be involuntary / Feels as though the urine will not come out / Urine tends to be suppressed or difficult to pass / Sediment in the urine looks like coffee grounds	**Heat, hot rooms, hot drinks, a hot bath, or lying under covers in bed** / Pressure / After sleep / Lying down / Exercise	**Cool air or cold bath or shower** / Uncovering / Motion / Sitting erect	Not thirsty / Crave sour
Cantharis *(Spanish fly)*	**Extreme symptoms** / **Very rapid onset of bladder symptoms** / **Intolerable pain** / **Bloody urine** / **Tremendous urgency and frequency**	In a frenzy / Restlessness	Intense stinging, cutting, and burning pain on urination / Urine is scalding and comes out drop by drop with intolerable pain / Constant desire to urinate / Strain tremendously to urinate / Fever and chills / Strong sexual desire	**Urinating** / Cold drinks / Hearing the sound of water	Rubbing / Rest / Warmth / Lying quietly on your back	Desire for wine
Mercurius corrosivus *(Mercuric chloride)*	**Tremendous urge to urinate** / **The urge to urinate is not relieved by urination** / **Urine is only passed drop by drop with great pain**	Anxious and restless / Difficulty thinking and speaking clearly / You don't understand what others say to you	Intense burning in the urethra / Urine is hot and burning / Bleeding of urethra after urination / Spasm of bladder and rectum / Blood in urine	Urination / Bowel movement	Rest	

78

Remedy	Symptoms	Mind	Worse	Better	Food
Sarsaparilla *(Wild licorice)* **Severe pain in the urethra at the end of urination** **Right-sided symptoms**	**Urine may be difficult to pass while sitting, only dribbling out** Can only urinate while standing Urine is scanty, slimy, flaky, sandy, or bloody Pain from the right kidney extending downward Gas released from the bladder during urination Bladder is tender and swollen	Anxious and depressed from the pain Easily offended	At night Yawning Motion Cold	Standing Uncovering the neck and chest	Eating bread and drinking water disagree with you
Staphysagria *(Stavesacre)* **"Honeymoon cystitis" (occurs following sexual intercourse)** **Toothaches, headaches**	**Desire to urinate but can't after sex with a new partner or during pregnancy** **Sensation of a drop of urine continuously rolling along the urethra** Burning in the urethra while urinating Urging and pain after urination Frequent urge to urinate results in a scanty or profuse discharge of watery urine	**Symptoms come on after suppressed anger, indignation, embarrassment, or insult** Mild personality Want to please	**Too much sex** Masturbation	Warmth Rest Expressing emotions	Desire for or aversion to milk Crave sweets, tobacco

Breastfeeding Problems (See also Mastitis)

Description

Over half of the women in the United States breastfeed their infants today and the number is growing. There is considerable evidence that breastfeeding increases the immunity of your baby as well as your maternal bond with your child. Your most common breastfeeding problems will likely be engorgement and inadequate milk production. Homeopathy is an excellent type of medicine for you if you nurse your baby, because conventional drugs pass into your breast milk and homeopathic medicines are totally safe.

Symptoms

Engorgement is characterized by swelling and discomfort of the breast and soreness of your nipples and generally occurs within the first few days after your baby is born, when the milk begins to come in. Inadequate milk production, which can be quite discouraging, means that either you do not have enough breast milk or that your milk dries up before you are ready to wean your baby. Excessive lactation means that you produce more milk than your baby needs.

Complications

The most serious complication of inadequate milk production, which is not supplemented in some other form, is the baby's failure to thrive and, in extreme cases, death.

Look

What is the color, appearance, and texture of my breast milk?
Is there any discoloration of my breast(s)?
Any swelling?
Anything unusual about the appearance of my nipples?
How much breast milk do I produce?
Does my baby seem to have any problem with my breast milk?

Listen

"I have way too much breast milk and my breasts are red, hot, swollen, and tender." *Belladonna*

"My breasts are engorged. They feel so painful every time I move!"
  Bryonia
"My milk is watery and tastes really bad! My baby refuses to drink it."
  Calcarea carbonica
"My breast milk stopped flowing when I got a cold." *Dulcamara*
"Help! I've only nursed for three months and my milk is drying up."
  Lac caninum
"My breasts are shrinking, my milk is drying up, but the rest of me feels
  so fat!" *Lac defloratum*
"My problem is milk all around. I don't drink it and I can't seem to pro-
  duce enough." *Lactuca virosa*
"My milk is thin and watery and has a bitter taste. I just cry every time I
  nurse my baby." *Pulsatilla*
"My nipples are inverted, I feel sharp pain in my breasts, and my breast
  milk is bloody." *Silica*
"I really need help getting my milk flow going. My only other complaint is
  horrendous hives." *Urtica urens*

Ask

When did I first begin to have problems breastfeeding my baby?
Did I have any illness just before my milk problems began?
Did I experience any emotional problems just before?
How do I feel about my difficulty breastfeeding?
Do I have any breast pain?
How does my milk taste?

Pointers for Finding Your Homeopathic Medicine

• If your breasts are hot, red, and painful with red streaks, take *Bel-
ladonna*.
• For breast pain that is worse with any motion and better remaining still,
Bryonia is best.
• *Calcarea carbonica* can help women with swollen breasts and profuse,
watery, bad-tasting milk.
• In the case of hard, sore, engorged breasts or suppression of milk follow-
ing a cold, take a look at *Dulcamara*.
• *Lac caninum* is an excellent medicine to dry up breast milk.
• *Lac defloratum* is very helpful to bring back milk when the flow has
stopped.

• A useful medicine to stimulate milk secretion in breasts that dry up is *Lactuca virosa*.

• If you are tenderhearted with little milk and changeable symptoms, think of *Pulsatilla*.

• If milk production is suppressed and the nipples are drawn in, consider *Silica*.

• For absence of milk production with no apparent cause, try *Urtica urens*.

Dosage

• Take three pellets of 30C every one to two hours until you see an improvement.

• If you are no better after three doses, change medicines.

• After you first notice you have improved, take another dose only if your symptoms begin to return.

• Lower potencies (6X, 6C, and 30X) may need to be given more often (every one to two hours, depending on the symptoms.

• Higher potencies (200X, 200C, and 1M) usually need to be taken only once but may need a repetition if the symptoms are severe or return after initial improvement.

What to Expect from Women's Homeopathic Self-Care

If engorgement is your problem, you should begin to notice less swelling and more ease of milk flow within a few days of starting homeopathy. Give each well-indicated medicine three to four days before making any changes. If your milk flow diminishes, the right homeopathic medicine should bring back your normal milk production within four to five days. Wait that long before you consider changing medicines. If the indicated medicine(s) here is not effective within ten days, seek out constitutional care from a homeopathic practitioner quickly so that you do not have to stop nursing your baby.

Women's Naturopathic Self-Care Recommendations

For engorgement:

• If you have flat or inverted nipples, wear breast shields during pregnancy to draw them out.

• Wear a comfortable nursing bra twenty-four hours a day for support.

- Express your milk manually while you take a hot shower and just before you nurse so that your baby can get his mouth comfortably around your areola.
- Reposition your baby during nursing.
- If your baby refuses to nurse, give your milk on a spoon rather than in a bottle. Do not give up easily on breastfeeding. Seek out advice if you are at your wit's end.
- Dry the milk on your nipples with a hairdryer on the low setting between feedings.
- Apply hot packs to your breasts just before nursing and cold packs just after.
- Contact La Leche League. They provide a wealth of information and support for nursing moms.

If you do not produce enough milk:

- Drink lots of water.
- Eat a healthful diet of whole, natural foods and eliminate caffeine and alcohol.
- Relax, de-stress, and visualize having plenty of breast milk to satisfy your baby.
- Alternate breasts during nursing.
- Feed your baby on demand.
- If you need to supplement your breast milk, use goat's milk or even soy milk, rather than cow's milk. Goat's milk is the closest in its content to mother's milk and is the least allergenic.

If you produce too much milk:

- If your milk flows too freely and quickly, express a small quantity prior to nursing.
- Adjust your baby's nursing position so that gravity assists in slowing your milk flow.
- Limiting your nursing to only one breast per feeding can decrease your milk production.
- Relax and know that your breast milk supply should normalize within a couple of months.

BREASTFEEDING PROBLEMS

	Key Symptoms	Mind	Body	Worse	Better	Food & Drink
Belladonna (Deadly nightshade)	Sudden onset Violent, intense symptoms Right-sided symptoms Inflammation	Flare-ups of anger Desire to escape Lively, vivacious	Breasts are hot, red, heavy, hard Red streaks across breasts Milk flow profuse, obstructed, or absent	Touch Being jarred Suppressed perspiration	Bed rest Lightly covering the breast	Desire for lemons or lemonade
Bryonia (Wild hops)	All symptoms are worse from motion Dryness of skin and mucous membranes Extremely irritable Worse at 9:00 P.M.	You are obsessed with work You just want to go home	Your breasts are hot, painful, and hard Lumpy breasts with diminished milk secretion You ache all over Bursting headache Your lips are dry and parched	Any motion Becoming irritated Becoming overheated	Pressure to painful breast Lying on painful breast Hot packs	You want large quantities of cold water
Calcarea carbonica (Calcium carbonate)	Chilly with a tendency to sweat Tendency to put on weight easily Overly responsible Cautious and protective of self and family	Strong need to protect loved ones Overwhelmed by too much to do Concerns about security Couch potato Fear of heights, mice	Excess production of watery milk Milk abundant or deficient Breasts are hot and swollen Your milk disagrees with the baby Lack of energy to produce milk	Exertion Becoming chilled Overwork	Dry climate Being warm	Love dairy products, especially cheese Desire for salty food
Dulcamara (Bitter-sweet)	Problems of the mucous membranes Symptoms that come on after exposure to cold, damp weather Sick from working in a damp environment	Strong-willed You tend to be controlling	Milk production absent or less since getting a cold Breasts are engorged, hard, sore	Cold, damp Becoming chilled Overwork	Warm, dry climate Motion	Aversion to food Great thirst for cold drinks
Lac caninum (Dog's milk)	Symptoms alternate from side to side Floating sensation Difficulty with nurturing or being nurtured	You think others look down on you Constant desire to wash your hands Dreams of snakes	Need to dry up breast milk Loss of milk production while nursing	Touch Being jarred	Open air	Desire for pepper, mustard, and pungent foods

Remedy					
Lac defloratum *(Skimmed milk)*	Violent headaches Intolerance of milk Chilly	Sense of rejection by your community Feel that you or your friends will die Claustrophobia	Emaciation or atrophy of your breast Can quickly restore milk production Extreme constipation	Touching cold things Milk	Rest Profuse urination	Allergy or aversion to milk
Lactuca virosa *(Wild lettuce)*	Sense of lightness of body as if swimming Tightness of whole body, especially chest Excellent medicine for stimulating milk production	Restlessness with fear and anxiety Can't remember what you wanted to say Disturbed sleep due to anxiety	No breast milk Tightness of your chest as if you would suffocate Sleepiness while having a bowel movement Cannot lie on your back	Touch Pressure Warm room	Outdoor exercise	Desire for milk You feel worse from drinking milk
Pulsatilla *(Windflower)*	Your symptoms change like the wind Highly emotional One of the most important homeopathic medicines for women Worse from becoming overheated	Easily brought to tears You are warm, affectionate, and love nurturing You need others around You cry while nursing your baby	Breast milk thin, watery, suppressed, blocked Milk flowing and profuse You produce milk even though you are not nursing	Warm room without ventilation Rich foods	Being outside Love and nurturing	Desire for fats Feel worse from fats
Silica *(Flint)*	Low stamina and energy Abscesses and glandular swellings Obstinate constipation Usually on the thin side	Refined High standards for yourself Must meet the standards of others Shy Proper and fastidious	Milk suppressed or absent Thin, bad-tasting milk that your baby refuses Nipples drawn in like a funnel Delicate features, like a porcelain doll	Cold draft Suppressed perspiration	Wrapping up	Worse from cold food and fats Desire for eggs
Urtica urens *(Stinging nettle)*	Stinging pain after burns or insect bites Nettle rash First- and second-degree burns or scalds Hives	Restless, nervous Difficult to think	No breast milk without apparent cause Swollen breasts	A cold bath	Rubbing the affected area	Allergic reaction to shellfish

Fear of Flying

Description
Fear of flying is the second most common type of phobia, after public speaking. The specific fear can vary from feeling an intense claustrophobia to feeling out of control or fearing that the plane will crash and you will die. This out-of-proportion concern can be debilitating to women who need to travel long distances and it keeps plane-phobia classes full.

Symptoms
Physical symptoms of fear of flying are like those of other phobias and panic attacks: tight muscles, heart palpitations, cold sweat, rapid pulse, and hyperventilation. These can occur either before flight, before the plane actually takes off, or while you are in the air. They can be provoked by turbulence during the flight.

Complications
Acute fear can induce fainting, shock, and, in rare cases, a heart attack.

Look
Look in the mirror. Do you appear frightened?
Are you hyperventilating?
Has the color of your face changed?
Are you sweating?
Trembling?

Listen
"I'm terrified that the plane will crash and we'll all die." *Aconite*
"I'm so afraid my plane will crash tomorrow and I'll die that I'm already pacing. If I only had company, I'd feel better." *Arsenicum album*
"What if the pilot falls asleep? Or gets food poisoning? Or has a heart attack? Just thinking about it gives me a lump in my throat." *Argentum nitricum*
"I feel really out of it for days after those scary landings." *Borax*
"I'll have to take care of everybody until we're safe and sound and back on the ground." *Calcarea carbonica*

Ask

Have I ever had fear of flying in the past?

What exactly am I afraid of?

How does thinking about flying in a plane make me feel?

What would make me feel more relaxed?

Am I hungry? For anything special? Thirsty?

Does anything make me feel better or worse?

Do I feel warm or chilly?

Does it help to be in any particular position?

Pointers for Finding Your Homeopathic Medicine

• If your fear of flying is sudden, extreme, precipitated by a frightening event, and punctuated by a strong fear of dying, take *Aconite*.

• When you find yourself pacing, unable to calm your anxiety before a flight, insecure, and much more concerned about your own well-being than about people around you, consider *Arsenicum album*.

• If your fear manifests itself in an impulsive quality and a tendency to think of every possible thing that might go wrong, *Argentum nitricum* is a likely bet.

• *Borax* can be helpful for sensitive travelers who startle easily and hate loud noise and plane landings.

• If you feel overwhelmed and overly responsible for making sure every-one around you is safe, think of *Calcarea carbonica*.

Dosage

• It often helps to take a dose of the indicated medicine the day before, the morning of, or just prior to the flight.

• Take three pellets of 30C every fifteen minutes until you see an improve-ment.

• If you are no better after three doses, change medicines.

• After you first notice you have improved, take another dose only if your symptoms begin to return.

• Lower potencies (6X, 6C, and 30X) may need to be given more often (every one to two hours, depending on the severity of the symptoms).

• Higher potencies (200X, 200C, and 1M) usually need to be taken only once but may need a repetition if the symptoms are severe or return after initial improvement.

What to Expect from Women's Homeopathic Self-Care

The correct homeopathic medicine should help you feel more relaxed within ten to fifteen minutes. Your anxiety will be considerably diminished so that you can put your mind on more important matters, like having a great time on your trip.

Women's Naturopathic Self-Care Recommendations

• Lie back in your seat, close your eyes, and take long, deep breaths.

• Visualize yourself having enjoyed your flight and having reached your destination safe and sound.

• Avoid drinking caffeine or alcohol on the flight. Instead, bring a relaxing herbal tea, such as chamomile, or purified water along with nutritious snacks.

• If you prefer to sit in a certain area of the plane, arrange it well in advance.

• Decrease your flying stress by being realistic about checked baggage and carry-on luggage, allowing plenty of time to get to the airport, and making any house-sitting, childcare, parking, or other arrangements ahead of time.

• Bring along a favorite book, laptop solitaire, letters, or whatever else it takes to absorb your concentration.

• Sharing your concerns with the passenger seated next to you, or just chatting with him or her, can sometimes be an excellent distraction.

• If you are without any homeopathic medicines, take Bach Flower Essence Rescue Remedy (five drops under the tongue every fifteen minutes).

	Key Symptoms	Mind	Body	Worse	Better	Food & Drink
Aconite (Monkshood)	Fear of airplanes and crowds Sudden fright and emotional shock about the airplane flight Very afraid of death or sure that you will die, even predicting the time when the plane will crash Extreme anxiety Tremendous restlessness	Anguish Claustrophobia (fear of enclosed or narrow places) Agoraphobia (fear of wide open spaces, leaving the house) Desire for the company of others	Rapid heartbeat and violent heart palpitations Profuse perspiration with anxiety Shortness of breath Flushing or paleness of the face Hot, heavy, burning sensation in the head	Chill	Fresh air Rest Wine	Strong thirst for lots of cold water
Argentum nitricum (Silver nitrate)	Anticipation, apprehension, and fear before the flight Fear of heights Feeling of being trapped (claustrophobia) during the flight Anxiety about getting to the plane on time	Impulse to jump out of the airplane Anxious	Bloated with gas Diarrhea from fear Sore throat and hoarseness	**Anxiety before an event** Crowds Heat Sugar	Cool air Open air	Desire for sweets, salty foods, cheese
Arsenicum album (Arsenic)	Tremendous anxiety before and during the flight Fear of dying in a plane crash Restlessness	Very anxious about health Insomnia after midnight, 1:00 to 2:00 A.M. Want to have company and fear being left alone Needy and demanding	Burning pains Very chilly Palpitations	Midnight to 2:00 A.M. Cold food or drinks	Heat Warm drinks	Want to sip cold drinks frequently Desire for milk, the fat on meat, sour food, and warm food
Borax (Sodium biborate)	Fear during descent Worse from downward motion of any kind Startle easily from noise Anxiety from travel	Fear that you will catch a contagious disease Very sensitive Capricious	Nausea, vomiting, diarrhea Dry mucous membranes Trembling, dizziness Canker sores	**Downward motion** **Sudden noises**	11:00 P.M.	Worse from fruit

continued on next page

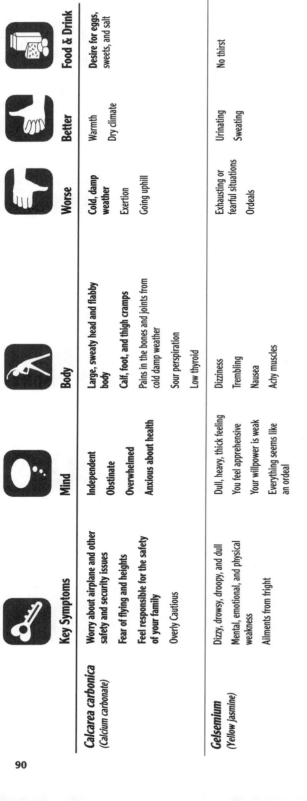

		Key Symptoms	Mind	Body	Worse	Better	Food & Drink
Calcarea carbonica (Calcium carbonate)		Worry about airplane and other safety and security issues	Independent	Large, sweaty head and flabby body	Cold, damp weather	Warmth	Desire for eggs, sweets, and salt
		Fear of flying and heights	Obstinate	Calf, foot, and thigh cramps	Exertion	Dry climate	
		Feel responsible for the safety of your family	Overwhelmed	Pains in the bones and joints from cold damp weather	Going uphill		
		Overly Cautious	Anxious about health	Sour perspiration			
				Low thyroid			
Gelsemium (Yellow jasmine)		Dizzy, drowsy, droopy, and dull	Dull, heavy, thick feeling	Dizziness	Exhausting or fearful situations	Urinating	No thirst
		Mental, emotional, and physical weakness	You feel apprehensive	Trembling	Ordeals	Sweating	
		Aliments from fright	Your willpower is weak	Nausea			
			Everything seems like an ordeal	Achy muscles			

Fright (Acute)

Description

Fright, or even terror, occurs when you experience a sudden shock or extreme fear, such as after you have witnessed horrible or frightening events like a car accident, earthquake, assault, or even a terrifying movie.

Symptoms

Immediately following the frightening experience, you may notice a rapid heartbeat, shortness of breath, shock, cold sweat, hyperventilation, trembling, diarrhea, nausea, dizziness, and, less often, fainting.

Complications

If such a condition persists long after the event, it may be diagnosed as post-traumatic stress syndrome. People who have suffered terrifying experiences may later develop panic attacks and, rarely, heart attacks, amnesia, or loss of speech or vision.

Look

Do I look scared?
Has my breathing changed?
Do I scream? Cry? Pace?
Has my mood changed significantly? If it has, in what way?
Do I have nightmares?

Listen

"We will have another earthquake tonight and I will die. I just know it."
   Aconite
"Every time I have to drive over a bridge, I just about lose it." *Argentum
   nitricum*
"I've been in a state of shock and fear ever since my car accident." *Arnica*
"I'm afraid someone will break into my house so I double-lock every-
   thing." *Arsenicum album*
"I feel terrified of going out alone in the dark because a wild animal might
   eat me." *Stramonium*

Ask

What brought on my fright in the first place?

What am I *most* afraid of?

Do any physical symptoms go along with the fear? What are they?

Does my acute fear prevent me from doing anything in my life? What?

Pointers for Finding Your Homeopathic Medicine

• The first medicine to think of for terror or fright is *Aconite*.

• If there is an exaggerated fear of high places, elevators, bridges, or losing control, consider *Argentum nitricum*.

• When the fright began during an accident or trauma, take a look at *Arnica*.

• If you feel anxiety and insecurity that is out of proportion to the situation, particularly a fear of being robbed, think about *Arsenicum album*.

• For terror of being alone, especially in the dark, with a strong desire to cling to someone else, *Stramonium* is a good possibility.

Dosage

• Take three pellets of 30C every fifteen minutes until you see an improvement.

• If you are no better after three doses, change medicines.

• After you first notice you have improved, take another dose only if your symptoms begin to return.

• Lower potencies (6X, 6C, and 30X) may need to be given more often (every one to two hours, depending on the intensity of the fear).

• Higher potencies (200X, 200C, and 1M) usually need to be taken only once, but may need a repetition if the symptoms are severe or return after initial improvement.

What to Expect from Women's Homeopathic Self-Care

If your fright is recent, you should except to see a significant improvement in a matter of hours or days. If the exaggerated fear does not dissipate within a month, or if you are suffering from fright that occurred months or years ago, seek the help of a qualified homeopathic practitioner because the likelihood of homeopathy helping you get over your fear is very high.

Women's Naturopathic Self-Care Recommendations

• Remind yourself that, regardless of what might have happened to you, you are now safe.

• Have a friend, family member, or someone else you can trust with you for a day or two.

• Put yourself in an environment in which you feel safe, secure, and comfortable.

• If you are still in any danger, seek medical, legal, or other help as appropriate.

• Do deep breathing and relaxation exercises.

• If you need counseling to talk about what happened to you, don't hesitate to seek it. Some short-term psychotherapy techniques such as rapid eye movement and thought field therapy as well as hypnotherapy can be particularly effective.

	Key Symptoms	Mind	Body	Worse	Better	Food & Drink
Aconite (Monkshood)	Sudden fright, fear, and emotional shock Very afraid of death or sure that you will die, even predicting the time of death Extreme anxiety, restlessness Illnesses after a fright Symptoms that come on suddenly	Terror-stricken Anguished Claustrophobic (afraid of enclosed or narrow places) Agoraphobic (afraid of wide open spaces, leaving the house) Afraid of crowds, airplanes	Rapid heartbeat and violent heart palpitations Shortness of breath Flushing or paleness of the face Hot, heavy, burning sensation in the head Profuse perspiration with anxiety	Chill	Fresh air Rest Wine	Strong thirst for lots of cold water
Argenticum nitricum (Silver nitrate)	Fear of bridges and elevators Fear of losing control You feel hurried and must walk fast Impulses to do strange things	Irrational worries Fear that you will fail Afraid if you pass a high building Fear of crowds	Warm Trembling Digestive upset from fright Splinterlike pains	Crowds Closed Rooms Suspense	Cool air	You love salty foods and cheese
Arnica (Leopard's bane)	Shock of any kind Fright due to traumatic injury Fear of crowds and public places	Want to be left alone; insist that nothing is wrong Fear being touched	Black and blue areas following injury Sore, bruised feeling anywhere in the body	Touch Overexertion	Lying down with the head low	
Arsenicum album (Arsenic)	Tremendous anxiety; anxious about health Fear of death Restlessness Fear of robbers	Insomnia after midnight or at 3:00 A.M. Hypochondriacal Fear of germs and contagion Want to have company and fear being left alone	Very chilly Burning pains Palpitations Heartburn	Midnight to 2:00 A.M. Cold food or drinks	Heat Warm drinks	Want to sip cold drinks frequently Desire milk, fat on meat, sour foods
Stramonium (Thorn apple)	Very frightened, like being alone in a dark jungle filled with wild animals or in a graveyard at night Fear of the dark, water, dogs Clingy	Fear of running water and bright objects such as mirrors Rage or violence if attacked, provoked Fear of animals, death, ghosts, and nightmares	Convulsions Heart palpitations	Darkness	Light Company Warmth	Great thirst Desire for sweets Aversion to water

Grief (Acute)

Description

Grief is an emotional response to loss and disappointment, such as the loss of a loved one, the breakup of a relationship, the loss of a job, or the experience of a deeply meaningful life transition.

Symptoms

If you are grieving, you may weep, sob, sigh, withdraw, or, on the other hand, all of your emotions may become frozen in unexpressed sadness.

Complications

If you are extremely grief-stricken and do not receive the help you need, you may become seriously depressed and even suicidal. If you have more than fleeting thoughts of ending your life, contact your local crisis team or mental health center.

Look

How do I look?

Has my appearance changed?

Have I lost weight?

Are my eyes red from crying?

Do I take care of myself? Eat? Bathe? Go to work? See people?

Listen

"Ever since I was fired from my job a week ago, I feel like a total failure. I have nothing to live for." *Aurum metallicum*

"My mother died a month ago and I can't think of anything else. I sob all the time." *Ignatia*

"Since my partner dumped me, I just lock myself in my room and listen to sad music." *Natrum muriaticum*

"The joy has gone out of my life. I seem to have lost all of my interest in anything." *Phosphoric acid*

Ask

How do I feel?

Do I want to be with other people or by myself?

Is my sleep normal?

Have I experienced any physical symptoms since I began to feel this way?

What would make me feel better or worse?

Do I need to call someone to be with me?

Do I feel so bad that I need to call a crisis team?

Pointers for Finding Your Homeopathic Medicine

- *Aurum metallicum* is the best medicine if you feel as if a dark cloud has enveloped you and you have lost all hope.
- *Ignatia* is the first medicine to think of for acute grief and loss, especially if you are sobbing and sighing and can't make yourself stop crying.
- If others' efforts to console you only make you feel worse and you just want to hole up in your room and read romance novels or listen to sad music, take *Natrum muriaticum.*
- For a state of total apathy in which nothing brings you joy or sparks any enthusiasm, a good medicine to think of is *Phosphoric acid.*

Dosage

- Take three pellets of 30C every one to two hours until you see an improvement.
- If you are no better after three doses, change medicines.
- After you first notice you have improved, take another dose only if your symptoms begin to return.
- Lower potencies (6X, 6C, and 30X) may need to be given more often (every one to two hours, depending on the severity of the emotional suffering).
- Higher potencies (200X, 200C, and 1M) usually need to be taken only once but may need a repetition if the symptoms are severe or return after initial improvement.

What to Expect

Homeopathic medicines can be extremely helpful for acute grief. The intense sadness and disappointment usually lessen to a significant degree within several days, sometimes within hours. If you are not better within a week or if your symptoms are severe or longstanding, find a homeopathic practitioner.

Women's Naturopathic Self-Care Recommendations

- Allow yourself to express your grief rather than holding it in.
- Find a shoulder to cry on.
- Stay as much as possible in the present moment rather than dwelling on the past.
- If your relationship has ended, release that person and move forward with your life.
- Find a psychotherapist who can help you process your grief and learn from it.
- Do something special for yourself.
- Do something special for someone else who needs your help.
- Try Bach Flower Essence Rescue Remedy.

	Key Symptoms	**Mind**	**Body**	**Worse**	**Better**	**Food & Drink**
Aurum metallicum (Gold)	Hopelessness Enveloped by a black cloud You feel you are a failure Disappointed love or business failure	No reason to go on Brooding melancholy Feeling that you have neglected your duty Sense of worthlessness Praying	Deep bone pains Heart palpitations Sinus problems	Alcohol Financial failure	Music	Loss of appetite
Ignatia (St. Ignatius bean)	Immediately following grief or loss Uncontrollable crying, loss of appetite, and extreme sadness Great mood swings Frequent sighing	High-strung and emotionally reactive Upset after hurt or disappointment Unpredictable and inconsistent	Numbness and cramping anywhere in the body Sensation of a lump in the throat A feeling of pressure or tightness in the chest Symptoms that are just the opposite of what you would expect	Disappointment	Deep breathing Changing positions	Strong desire for or dislike of fruit Desire for cheese
Natrum muriaticum (Sodium chloride)	Grief or disappointment in relationships Withdraw and isolate yourself after grief Feelings hurt very easily Hold back your tears	Very sensitive to the slightest reprimand or insult Pouty, sulky Deeply affected by music	Say you'll never be in a relationship again Introspective Headaches, canker sores, asthma, or herpes that began after a grief	10:00 A.M. Heat In the sunlight By the ocean	Open air	Desire for salty food, pasta, bread, and lemons Aversion to slimy food
Phosphoric acid	Exhaustion and apathy from grief, emotional shock, sudden loss or disappointed love Strong desire for large quantities of cold or carbonated beverages	Depressed Withdrawn Homesick	Extremely tired and burned out Painless diarrhea after grief Diarrhea doesn't cause exhaustion	Bad news Dehydration from loss of body fluids due to bleeding, diarrhea, and vomiting Cold	Warmth Naps	Desire for fruit, refreshing food, and carbonated drinks

Hemorrhoids

Description

Hemorrhoids, common to women, are varicose veins of the rectum. These veins may be located inside the rectum or they may protrude externally through the anus. The most common causes are constipation, pregnancy, and sitting for extended periods of time, although hemorrhoids may also be associated with liver problems.

Symptoms

Inflammation causes pain in the area of the hemorrhoids, varying in degree from mild to severe, which is the most bothersome symptom. You may also experience itching or bleeding. If you have a bad case of hemorrhoids, having a bowel movement or sitting may be excruciating.

Complications

Hemorrhoids can ulcerate and bleed profusely and, therefore, can be confused with colitis, colon polyps, or tumors. Blood clots may become lodged in the veins surrounding the hemorrhoid.

Look

Can I see my hemorrhoids, or can someone take a look at them for me?
What color are they?
Is there one hemorrhoid or several?
What is the extent of the swelling?
In there blood in my stool?
Do I hold myself in any particular position?

Listen

"My hemorrhoids are purple. The only time I feel relief from the pain is after they bleed." *Aesculus*
"I feel a sticking pain in my rectum when my hemorrhoids flare up." *Aesculus* and *Collinsonia*
"My stool is pure mucus." *Aloe*
"My hemorrhoids are so swollen and they bleed profusely." *Hamamelis*
"The hemorrhoids come when I get really constipated, drink wine, or worry too much about business." *Nux vomica*

"The part I hate the most about my hemorrhoids is how much my rectum itches." *Sulphur*

Ask

When did my hemorrhoids begin?

Was there any particular cause?

What bothers me the most about them?

How would I describe the pain or sensation? How intense is it?

When does the pain occur?

What makes it better or worse?

Have my bowel movements changed since the hemorrhoids flared up?

Have any other physical symptoms cropped up since the hemorrhoids came?

Have I experienced any mental and emotional changes or stress that led up to the hemorrhoids or that I feel since they came?

Pointers for Finding Your Homeopathic Medicine

• If your main symptom is rectal pain that feels like small sticks, consider *Aesculus* and *Collinsonia*.

• If swelling and bleeding are prominent, think first of *Hamamelis*.

• If you feel chilly, overstressed, have been drinking too much, and worry too much about your work, you may need *Nux vomica*.

• If you are warm-blooded and have lots of rectal itching that is worse in bed or after a hot shower or bath, *Sulphur* will often work.

Dosage

• Take three pellets of 30C every three to four hours until you see an improvement.

• If you are no better after three doses, change medicines.

• After you first notice you have improved, take another dose only if your symptoms begin to return.

• Lower potencies (6X, 6C, and 30X) may need to be given more often (every one to two hours, depending on the severity of the hemorrhoids).

• Higher potencies (200X, 200C, and 1M) usually need to be taken only once but may need a repetition if the symptoms are severe or return after initial improvement.

What to Expect

You should feel better within one to four days after taking the correct medicine. If your hemorrhoids are chronic, consult a homeopath for constitutional care.

Women's Naturopathic Self-Care Recommendations

- Take a sitz bath. Fill the tub with hot water up to two inches below your navel. Sit with your knees bent. Stay in the tub for five minutes. Then squat in a tub of cold water for one minute. Repeat the cycle two to three times.
- Take 1,000 milligrams of bioflavonoids daily to strengthen your capillaries.
- Be sure to keep your rectal area clean.
- If you are constipated, drink at least six glasses of water a day and take one tablespoon of bran, ground flaxseed or flaxseed oil, or psyllium seed once to twice daily until the constipation is relieved.
- Avoid spicy foods if they seem to aggravate your hemorrhoids.
- Use homeopathic rectal astringent suppositories. They contain one or more of the medicines listed in the chart that follows.
- If your hemorrhoids are due to constipation, one to two glycerin rectal suppositories a day may be helpful.
- Witch hazel applied externally to the hemorrhoids is an excellent astringent and can help them to shrink.

Note: Hemorrhoids are one of the few conditions for which homeopathic suppositories or ointments (often containing several medicines) can be just as beneficial as oral medications.

	Key Symptoms	Mind	Body	Worse	Better	Food & Drink
Aesculus (Horse chestnut)	**Feel better when the hemorrhoids are bleeding**	Gloomy	**Pain persists long after having a bowel movement**	**After urination or stool**	Cool, open air	Aversion to food in general
	Hemorrhoids are external, purple, and painful	Irritable	Stools are dry, hard, and knotty	During sleep	Bathing	
	Rectum feels full of small sticks	Confused and bewildered upon awakening	Burning in the anus	tea		
			Chills and sharp, shooting pains up the back			
Aloe (Aloe socotrina)	**Feeling of insecurity in the rectum as though stool would come out**	Irritable, discontented, and angry, with abdominal pain or constipation	**Hemorrhoids are filled with blood and feel congested**	Heat and summer	Cool, open air, cold bathing, and cold applications	Desires beer
	Hemorrhoids like a bunch of grapes	Don't want to be around people	**Stool comes out while passing gas**	Hot damp weather	Passing gas	
	Stools contain gelatinous lumps of mucus		Rumbling and gurgling in bowels, with sudden, gushing watery stool	After eating or drinking		
			Gushing stool is worse early morning in bed	Beer		
			Diarrhea after beer or oysters			
Collinsonia (Stone-root)	**Sensation of sharp sticks or sand in the rectum**	**Ailments from emotional excitement**	**Hemorrhoids are painful and bleed**	Cold	Warmth	Desire for or aversion to cheese
	Hemorrhoids combined with heart palpitations or constricted feeling in the heart	**Excited, with heart palpitations**	**Chronic constipation alternating with diarrhea**	Pregnancy	Morning	
	Hemorrhoids with swelling of the face or lips	Indecisive	Heaviness in rectum			
			Anus itches and may prolapse			
Hamamelis (Witch hazel)	Weakness of veins leading to congestive fullness, bleeding, and a sore, bruised feeling	Irritable	**Throbbing in the rectum**	Injuries	Rest	Aversion to water
	Hemorrhoids are swollen, purple, and filled with blood	Feel peaceful despite bleeding	**Pain often lasts for hours after a bowel movement**	Pressure or touch		
	Hemorrhoids and nosebleeds may occur together		**Considerable bleeding**			
			Anus feels sore, raw, and as if full of sticks			
			Back pain; sharp shooting pains up the back or into the sacroiliac joints or hips			
			Burning and chills up and down the back			

Nux vomica (*Quaker's button*)	**Hemorrhoids after too much stress, rich food, drugs, alcohol, or stimulants** **Hemorrhoids from chronic constipation** **Unsuccessful efforts to have a stool, with great urging and straining**	**Irritable** **Impatient** **Type A personality** Competitive and hard-driving Easily offended Frustrated easily by little things	**Itching, painful hemorrhoids** **May not even have the urge for a bowel movement** **Rectum feels constricted** May also have indigestion and heartburn Wake with pain or discomfort at 3:00 A.M.	Cold, drafts Rich foods, high living **Sedentary lifestyle** **Coffee and other stimulants** Pressure of clothing	Warmth Hot drinks After stool	Desire for stimulants, rich food, and fat
Sulphur	**Hemorrhoids both internal and external** **Very large hemorrhoids, in bunches** **Hemorrhoids itching, tender, and bleeding** **Rectal itching**	**Opinionated and critical** **Thinking all the time, philosophical** **Lazy** Usually messy, but sometimes very neat	**Diarrhea drives you out of bed in the morning around 5:00 A.M.** **Anus is red, sore, raw, burning, and very itchy** Stool is loose and burning Spasms in the rectum Bad-smelling sweat and vaginal area	**Warmth, and warmth of bed** **Bathing in warm water** Left side	Open air Sweating	Desire for alcohol, sweets, and spicy foods Aversion to eggs

103

Hot Flashes

Description

Hot flashes or flushes are brief episodes of heat, often accompanied by perspiration and followed by chills, that come during menopause in approximately 75 percent of women. They may be transient or, in the case of about one quarter of women, last five years or longer. The onset of menopause occurs most typically around age fifty-one; however, age of onset varies. Hot flashes also occur following a hysterectomy at any age.

Symptoms

You first feel warm or hot, then usually your face and neck become red and you perspire, sometimes profusely. The flash generally lasts from several seconds to five minutes and is followed by chills. This sequence is likely to make you throw off extra clothing or covers, then put them back on when you become chilled. You may also experience a variety of other symptoms during menopause. (See Menopause in chapter 13.)

Complications

Hot flashes can be annoying, embarrassing, or, at their worst, debilitating, especially if your sleep is significantly interrupted.

Look

Does my coloring change when I experience a hot flash?
Do I perspire? Where? How much?
Do I need to remove or add clothing or covers?
Do I have any other noticeable symptoms?

Listen

"I have hot flashes and I feel like I'm losing my mind." *Cimicifuga*
"I just want to scream and I can't stand anything tight around my neck."
    Lachesis
"I can't live with myself because I'm such a cry baby." *Pulsatilla*
"My skin is hot and dry and I'm burning up." *Sanguinaria*
"Just leave me alone and forget about sex!" *Sepia*
"My skin itches all over." *Sulphur*

Ask

When did my hot flashes begin?

Do I still get periods? If not, when was my last period?

What bothers me most about my hot flashes?

How intense are they?

What makes them better or worse?

Have any other physical symptoms begun along with the hot flashes?

How do I feel mentally and emotionally?

Pointers for Finding Your Homeopathic Medicine

- If your joints ache and you sigh all the time, consider *Cimicifuga*.
- One of the most common medicines for hot flashes, especially if you are on the verge of "exploding," is *Lachesis*.
- If you've had a history of hormonal problems with moodiness, you cry easily, and you hate getting too hot, *Pulsatilla* is a good bet.
- *Sanguinaria* can be quite helpful if you have dry mucous membranes, especially along with right shoulder pain.
- *Sepia* is the number one medicine for hot flashes if your sexual energy is diminished and you are constipated and grouchy.
- If your hot flashes are worse in bed or after a hot bath, you're itchier than usual, and you want to stick your feet out from under the covers, think of *Sulphur*.

Dosage

- Take three pellets of 30C once a day until you see an improvement.
- If you are no better after three doses, change medicines.
- After you first notice you have improved, take another dose only if your symptoms begin to return.
- Lower potencies (6X, 6C, and 30X) may need to be given more often (every one to two hours, depending on the severity of the hot flashes).
- Higher potencies (200X, 200C, and 1M) usually need to be taken only once but may need a repetition if the symptoms are severe or return after initial improvement.

What to Expect

You should feel better within one week of taking the correct medicine. If this does not occur or you have tried two or three medicines, see a homeopath, preferably before starting hormone therapy. A note of caution: Do not take homeopathic *Lachesis* more than twice daily for a week, or less frequently for longer than a month, without professional guidance because, in some sensitive women, a proving can occur. (In a proving you begin to develop symptoms of *Lachesis* that you don't already have.) If this happens, stop taking the medicine and consult a homeopath.

Women's Naturopathic Self-Care Recommendations

- Avoid or minimize hot, spicy, or hot-temperature foods.
- Wear loose clothing and layers that you can comfortably remove and add back on.
- Menopausal herbal formulas containing black cohosh, chasteberry, and dong quai can be very helpful.
- Promensil, a product containing red clover, may alleviate hot flashes.
- One thousand milligrams a day of hesperidin, a bioflavonoid, can reduce hot flashes.
- Boron, a trace mineral, can reduce hot flashes as well as decrease your risk of osteoporosis.
- Many women find natural estrogen and progesterone creams containing wild yam to be very useful.
- A diet high in soy and flax is recommended.
- Take vitamin E, 800 milligrams a day, unless you have high blood pressure.
- Avoid smoking and drinking.
- Drink lots of water.

	Key Symptoms	Mind	Body	Worse	Better	Food & Drink
Cimicifuga (Black cohosh)	Crampy muscle pains Intense gloominess Nervousness and agitation	Feeling of a black cloud over you Fear you are going crazy Sighing Fear of mice	Heaviness in the extremities Pelvic pain from hip to hip Stiffness and tension in the neck and back	Cold, damp air Motion	Rest Wrapping up	Worse from alcohol
Lachesis (Bushmaster snake)	Symptoms are worse on left side of your body Symptoms move from left side to right You feel worse after sleep or on waking Intense symptoms and personality	Feel as if you will explode Jealous and suspicious Very talkative Fear of snakes	Prominent medicine for hot flashes if mental and emotional symptoms match You can't stand tight clothing around your neck or abdomen Can't bear for the sheet to touch you at night Premenstrual anger gets better when your period begins	After sleep Constriction of any kind Suppression of emotions or symptoms	Physical or emotional discharge	Desire for coffee Desire for oysters Worse from coffee during menopause
Pulsatilla (Windflower)	Changeable moods and symptoms You cry extremely easily You feel much worse in a hot, stuffy room Want to be outside in the open air	Feelings of abandonment You want others around Have difficulty making decisions Sweet, affectionate, sensitive	Very quick to become overheated Tend to be round-bodied Hot flashes with puffy hands, feet, abdomen You blush easily	Heat Rich foods	Opening a window Taking a slow walk outdoors	Desire for fats and rich foods Aggravation from rich foods
Sanguinaria (Blood-root)	Congestion of blood to your head, chest, abdomen Symptoms are more right-sided Burning sensations Warm-blooded	Grumbly Feeling of dread	Red cheeks Burning pain in your palms and soles Right shoulder pain Dry mucous membranes Throbbing sensation	Menopause Sun	Lying on your back	Craving for spicy and pungent food

continued on next page

107

	Key Symptoms	Mind	Body	Worse	Better	Food & Drink
Sepia *(Cuttlefish ink)*	Hormonal problems of any kind You don't want to make love You love vigorous exercise or dancing Desire for vinegar, pickles, and other sour foods	Snappy, weepy Indifference or aversion to your family Feeling stuck, unmotivated, trapped You would rather be left alone	Sudden flushes of heat with weakness and sweat Sex is painful from dryness of your vagina and vulva Yellowish-green or white, foul-smelling vaginal discharge Lots of vaginal itching	4 to 6 P.M. Cold air	Vigorous exercise Dancing	Craving for vinegar and pickles Desire for chocolate
Sulphur	Hot-blooded Burning pains anywhere in the body Burning in the soles of your feet Independent, opinionated, messy	You think your way is best Critical Mechanically minded Full of creative ideas and plans	Hot flashes followed by chilliness Your hot flashes are worse at night in bed You feel hotter after a hot bath or shower Your feet become unbearably hot and you must uncover them Heat	Heat 11:00 A.M. After taking a hot bath or shower	Cooling off	Desire for sweets; spicy, fatty foods; alcohol Aversion to eggs

Insomnia

Description

If you have insomnia, you have difficulty either falling asleep, staying asleep, or feeling rested on waking. Your sleep problems may be caused by a variety of factors, including emotional distress, worrying too much, an overactive or upsetting dream life, hormones, pain, caffeine, the side effects of prescription drugs, overeating or eating too close to bedtime, or an environment that is not conducive to rest.

Symptoms

You may not be able to fall asleep at night, may sleep very lightly, may awaken frequently during the night, or may wake up very early in the morning. The result, in any case, is that you feel fatigued, or even exhausted, much or most of the time. Your dream life may also be disrupted. Poor sleep can contribute to a variety of other problems, such as irritability, stress, difficulty with academic or work performance, relationships, anxiety, and depression.

Complications

Your losing an occasional night of sleep may not make a great impact on your life, but if it continues night after night, it may well impair the quality of your life. Sleep deprivation over time can result in decreased alertness, clarity, patience, and overall health and well-being.

Look

Do I appear tired?
Do I have circles under my eyes? A dragged-out look?
Am I missing my usual perky, vigorous demeanor?

Listen

"I can't sleep ever since I woke up in the middle of the night during an earthquake." *Aconite*
"I wake up and start thinking about how my people are ripping me off." *Arsenicum album*
"My mind is so busy and full of daydreams and night dreams that I can't turn it off." *Coffea*

"My pain keeps me up." *Coffea, Chamomilla*

"I am so afraid I will blow my performance tomorrow that I can't get a wink of sleep." *Gelsemium*

"Ever since my cat ran away, I just can't sleep. I feel devastated that she's gone." *Ignatia*

"I have to win that tennis championship or else. Forget sleep!" *Nux vomica*

Ask

Do I just have occasional sleep problems or is it an ongoing problem?

What are my specific sleep problems?

Do I wake up consistently at a particular time?

Do any physical problems disrupt my sleep?

Is there some mental or emotional reason for my insomnia?

Have any physical problems started along with the sleep problems?

Do any factors like light or noise prevent me from sleeping well?

Do I, or does someone I sleep with, snore?

Does my eating affect my sleep in any way?

Do I prefer sleeping in a particular position?

Pointers for Finding Your Homeopathic Medicine

• If you can't sleep ever since you had a terribly frightening experience, take *Aconite*.

• For insomnia that began when you felt you were being robbed or cheated or your finances were in danger, consider *Arsenicum album*.

• If you jolt up in bed, wide awake at 3:00 A.M. with your mind full of ideas, take a look at *Coffea*.

• For sleeplessness due to hypersensitivity to pain, *Coffea* or *Chamomilla* can be very helpful.

• If the insomnia is due to performance anxiety, *Gelsemium* is a good bet.

• If your sleep problems were preceded by grief or the death of a loved one, think of *Ignatia*.

• If you wake in the middle of the night, usually around 3:00 A.M., with thoughts about how you can be more successful in business, look at *Nux vomica*.

Dosage

• Take three pellets of 30C every one to two hours until you see an improvement.

- If you are no better after three doses, change medicines.
- After you first notice you have improved, take another dose only if your symptoms begin to return.
- Lower potencies (6X, 6C, and 30X) may need to be given more often (every one to two hours, depending on the severity of the sleeplessness).
- Higher potencies (200X, 200C, and 1M) usually need to be taken only once but may need a repetition if the symptoms are severe or return after initial improvement.

What to Expect

If your sleep problem began recently, there is a good chance that you can help yourself by following these guidelines. In this case, you should notice improvement within a week. If it is a more long-standing problem, consult an experienced homeopathic practitioner.

Women's Naturopathic Self-Care Recommendations

- Drink a cup of warm milk (which contains the amino acid tryptophan) or a cup of chamomile tea one-half hour before bedtime.
- Equal parts of valerian root, skullcap, passionflower, and hops can be a useful herbal sedative. Take thirty drops of tincture in warm water one-half hour before bedtime or every two hours during the night as needed, up to three doses.
- Make the hour before you retire at night a time for quiet, relaxation, soft music, or inspirational reading.
- Lie on your right side with your arm outstretched to fall asleep more quickly. This position allows you to breathe through your left nostril, which is considered more calming.
- Alternating nostril breathing just before bedtime can be extremely beneficial. Close off your right nostril with your right thumb pressed against the side of your nose. Inhale slowly through your left nostril. With your middle finger, close off your left nostril, release your thumb to open your right nostril, and exhale. Inhale through the right nostril. Now close off the right nostril and exhale through the left. Inhale slowly through the left and switch again, exhaling through the right. Continue for three to ten minutes.

	Key Symptoms	Mind	Body	Worse	Better	Food & Drink
Aconite (Monkshood)	Insomnia due to fright or shock Extreme anxiety Tremendous restlessness Fear of impending death	Claustrophobia Panic attacks Want company	**Violent heart palpitations** **Profuse perspiration with anxiety** **Rapid pulse**	Lying on your side during your period	Fresh air Calming influences	Very thirsty for cold drinks
Arsenicum album (Arsenic)	Insomnia due to worry and anxiety Insomnia worse from midnight to 2:00 A.M. Restlessness	Very anxious about health Hypochondriacal Want someone close by for support Insomnia makes you more anxious Dream about worries and fears	**Burning pains** **Very chilly** Weakness and weight loss	After midnight Financial concerns Getting cold	Lots of covers Lying with head propped up	Desire for sips of water frequently Desire for milk
Chamomilla (Chamomile)	Looking for a fight Tremendous hypersensitivity to pain Symptoms worse after anger	Capricious Nothing makes you happy Rude	Excruciating menstrual pain Vomiting Profuse, dark, clotted menstrual flow	Cold wind Night 9:00 P.M.	Being carried	**Desire for cold water, sour drinks** **Aversion to and worse from coffee**
Coffea (Unroasted coffee)	Insomnia; wide awake at 3:00 A.M. with mind full of thoughts Overstimulation, hypersensitivity, and hyperexcitability Nervous agitation and restlessness	Unusual activity of body and mind Overreaction to all emotions, even joy and surprise Abundance of ideas Daydreaming	Exquisite sensitivity to pain Hypersensitivity to noise, light, and touch High sexual energy Insomnia or hot flashes during menopause	**Excessive emotions, including joy** Strong odors Noise Touch	Lying down Sleep	Aversion to and worse from coffee Aggravation from wine

Remedy	Insomnia indications	Mental/emotional	Physical symptoms	Causes	Worse from	Cravings/better
Gelsemium (*Yellow jasmine*)	**Insomnia following fright or from stage fright** / **Want to lie down and go to sleep, but can't** / **Diarrhea from stage fright** / **Dizzy, drowsy, and dull**	Mind feels extremely dull / Thinking is an effort		**Fright** / Shock	Bending forward / Lying down with the head up	Lack of thirst / Better from alcohol
Ignatia (*St. Ignatius bean*)	**Insomnia following grief or loss** / **Uncontrollable crying, loss of appetite, and extreme sadness** / **Pronounced mood swings**	High-strung and emotionally reactive / Upset after hurt or disappointment	**Frequent sighing** / **Numbness and cramping anywhere in the body** / Sensation of a lump in the throat, especially after grief / Symptoms that are just the opposite of what you would expect, such as an injury with no pain or feeling cold in a hot room	**Disappointment or humiliation** / Shock	Deep breathing / Changing positions	**Strong desire for or dislike for fruit** / Desire for cheese
Nux vomica (*Quaker's button*)	**Waking at 3:00 A.M. with thoughts of business** / **Highly irritable and impatient** / **Chilly**	**Obsessed with business** / **Want to be the first and the best** / **Competitive and hard-driving, Type A** / Easily offended / Frustrated easily by little things	**Insomnia due to heightened sensitivity to light, noise, sound, and other stimuli** / **Insomnia after too much rich or spicy food or alcohol**	**Hunger** / **Disappointed ambition** / Early morning	Naps / Lying on your side	**Desire for spicy food, fat, coffee, alcohol, and tobacco**

113

Jet Lag

Description

If you have ever flown across the world, or even the United States, you will likely be familiar with jet lag. It is the fatigue, disorientation, and stress induced by rapid travel across a number of time zones. This can be a serious problem for business travelers or intercontinental commuters.

Symptoms

Tiredness and insomnia are two of the most common characteristics of women who are jet-lagged; however, additional symptoms include anxiety (see Fear of Flying), a feeling of sadness or isolation, confusion, nausea (see Motion Sickness), rapid heart rate, and susceptibility to upper respiratory infections and other airborne-transmitted acute illnesses.

Complications

Chronic fatigue syndrome, thrombophlebitis, and dehydration may result from prolonged and untreated jet lag.

Look

Do I appear tired?
Do I have circles under my eyes? A dragged-out look?
Is my energy level normal?

Listen

"Every time I travel, I get terribly constipated and dehydrated." *Alumina*
"My body has taken quite a beating." *Arnica*
"Those trips to Europe and Asia disrupt my sleep for weeks." *Cocculus*
"I feel so wiped out that I can barely keep my eyes open." *Gelsemium*
"When I travel, first I get diarrhea, then hemorrhoids, then I'm wiped out." *Nitric acid*
"My skin gets so dry and cracked when I fly, especially in the winter." *Petroleum*

Ask

How long does it take me to recover from long flights?
Which physical symptoms bother me the most?

How is my sleep the week or two after I fly?
Does flying affect me mentally or emotionally?
Are my nerves affected by long-distance travel?
Does anything make my jet lag better or worse?

Pointers for Finding Your Homeopathic Medicine

- For jet lag in which the main symptoms are dehydration and constipation, consider *Alumina*.
- For muscle soreness and achiness, use *Arnica*.
- If the main symptom is anxiety, with pacing and fear of death, look at *Arsenicum*.
- If you feel exhausted, wrung out, and sleepless after flying, *Cocculus* may be of benefit.
- If you're dizzy, drowsy, droopy, and dull, try *Gelsemium*.
- *Petroleum* is the first medicine to think of for dehydration with dry, cracked skin from too much air travel.

Dosage

- Take three pellets of 30C every three to four hours until you see an improvement.
- If you are no better after three doses, change medicines.
- After you first notice you have improved, take another dose only if your symptoms begin to return.
- Lower potencies (6X, 6C, and 30X) may need to be given more often (every one to two hours, depending on the severity of the jet lag).
- Higher potencies (200X, 200C, and 1M) usually need to be taken only once but may need a repetition if the symptoms are severe or return after initial improvement.

What to Expect

You should feel better within three to six hours of taking the correct medicine. You may need to repeat it if the feeling of jet lag recurs on your future trips.

Women's Naturopathic Self-Care Recommendations

- Build in a period of at least eight to twelve hours of rest after arriving at your destination.

• Try to arrive and return on a Saturday so you have Sunday to relax and recover.

• Plan your trips to include down time, or you will need a vacation after your vacation.

• For long trips, consider upgrading to business or first class so you can stretch out and rest comfortably.

• Ease your way into a high-protein, low-calorie diet before traveling and continue it during your trip.

• Minimize sugar, caffeine, and alcohol on the airplane.

• Get up to stretch whenever possible and continue your exercise routine during your trip.

• Drink lots of water on the plane and throughout your travels.

• Lubricate your skin with soothing creams or oils.

• If airplane travel makes you gassy and constipated, drink more liquids; avoid beans, broccoli, and cauliflower; and eat more cooked vegetables.

• Some women wear a small deionizer around their necks to recycle the air in their immediate vicinity.

• Homeopathic No-Jet Lag is a combination homeopathic medicine that may be helpful.

	Key Symptoms	Mind	Body	Worse	Better	Food & Drink
Alumina (Aluminum)	Confusion and disorientation Feeling of having lost your identity or sense of self Severe constipation Very dehydrated	Time passes slowly—an hour seems like a day Weakness of memory and concentration Everything seems unreal You answer questions slowly and vaguely	Skin dried up and wrinkled No desire to have a bowel movement Straining during bowel movement You want to lie down, but that increases the fatigue	Morning or on waking	Damp weather	You desire potatoes or feel bad after eating them
Arnica (Leopard's bane)	Muscles are sore and achy Waking fitfully from sleep Overexertion	You say you are just fine Refuse help from others Prefer being alone You exaggerate your symptoms	Sore and achy after sleep Bruising Oversensitivity of your entire body	Sleep Overexertion Touch	Stretching out Changing position Fresh air	Craving for vinegar Intense thirst, but you don't know for what Lose your taste for milk and meat
Cocculus (Indian cockle)	Sick after caring for others Motion sickness, airsickness, seasickness Confusion and disorientation Severe constipation	Weakness after loss of sleep or caring for a loved one Nervous exhaustion Take a long time to gather your thoughts Lose your train of thought easily	Dizziness worse from looking at moving objects or out of a moving vehicle Nausea from dizziness Nausea from thinking about or smelling food	Traveling Loss of sleep	Sitting Lying on your side	Aversion to food
Petroleum (Coal oil)	Severely dry skin to the point of cracking and bleeding Sense of confusion or disorientation Bad-smelling perspiration	Easily lost and confused You get lost in familiar places Difficulty making a decision Argumentative	Ragged, chapped, cracked fingertips and heels Heartburn You have to get up at night to eat	Travel Cold weather	Dry weather Warm air	You crave beer Aversion to meat, fats, and cooked or hot foods

Labor and Delivery

Description

Labor, which usually occurs within three weeks before or after the expected date of delivery, includes various progressive events, beginning with the show (a significant amount of clear, thick, blood-tinged mucus); the breaking of water; and regular, intense contractions followed by three stages of transition. Many situations and symptoms can present themselves and I have included only the eight medicines most likely to meet your needs during delivery. Consult the Recommended Reading section in the appendix for further information.

Symptoms

Some of the more common physical symptoms of labor include moderate and brief to excruciating and persistent pain, minimal to excessive bleeding, tearing during delivery, failure of the cervix to dilate, and exhaustion. Mental and emotional symptoms are varied, but your feelings can range from terror and anger to elation and relief and can change very quickly during the various stages of your labor.

Complications

There are many complications of labor, including prolonged failure to dilate, prolonged labor, premature birth, the cord wrapped around the baby's neck, meconium aspiration, retained placenta, and postpartum hemorrhage. Whether or not there are complications, homeopathy is an *adjunct* to the care of your obstetrician, midwife, and other skilled health professionals and birth team members, either at the hospital, home, or a birthing center.

Look

How is your facial color and expression?

Observe the rhythm of your breathing and contractions.

What position(s) make you feel more comfortable and reduce your pain and discomfort?

Do you have a vaginal discharge of any kind and, if so, what is its appearance?

Are there any other observable features or symptoms?

Listen

"I feel terrified that I will die." *Aconite*

"I'm in shock." *Arnica*

"Help me! My labor's just not progressing." *Caulophyllum*

"I'm thoroughly exhausted after losing so much blood." *China*

"I'm going crazy." *Cimicifuga*

"I'm just too tired to push!" *Gelsemium*

"Hold my hand. Don't leave my side for a minute!" *Pulsatilla*

"Tell my husband to wait outside until the baby is born." *Sepia*

Ask

How am I doing?

How is my energy?

Which are my most intense physical symptoms?

Is my pain tolerable?

What are the specific features of my pain or other symptoms?

What makes my symptoms better or worse?

Could I use the help of a homeopathic medicine?

What is my emotional state?

What do I need right now to help me through this stage of labor?

Pointers for Finding Your Homeopathic Medicine

• The best homeopathic medicine for extreme fear of death is *Aconite*.

• *Arnica* is an excellent medicine for trauma, shock, and bleeding, can be used for exhaustion during labor, and is sometimes taken routinely following labor.

• *Caulophyllum* is an excellent medicine for stalled labor.

• If you feel weak after losing blood, *China* can be of great benefit.

• *Cimicifuga* can be a great aid for women with late labor, with cramps in the hips, or with pelvic pain from one side to the other.

• If you feel sleepy, exhausted, and can't keep your eyes open during labor, try *Gelsemium*.

• To speed up the birth of an overdue baby, try *Pulsatilla*.

• *Sepia*, among countless indications, is good for exhausted women who feel like moving around and exercising during labor.

Dosage

• Take three pellets of 30C every five minutes to four hours, depending on the situation, until you see an improvement.

- If you are no better after three doses, change medicines.
- After you first notice you have improved, take another dose only if your symptoms begin to return.
- Lower potencies (6X, 6C, and 30X) may need to be given more often (every one to two hours, depending on the severity of the symptoms).
- Higher potencies (200X, 200C, and 1M) usually need to be taken only once but may need a repetition if the symptoms are severe or return after initial improvement.

What to Expect

Homeopathy can produce a rapid and dramatic amelioration of symptoms during labor and can reestablish as normal a course of labor as possible given the specific circumstances.

During labor, you should expect symptoms to improve noticeably within ten minutes. Self-prescribe only for clear-cut and relatively minor symptoms during labor and delivery and only with the cooperation of your obstetrician or midwife. If your symptoms are severe or complex or if you have any sense at all that you are in over your head, consult an experienced prescriber or forget about using homeopathy and rely on your conventional practitioners. An emergency situation such as childbirth is not the ideal time to try homeopathy for the first time.

Women's Naturopathic Self-Care Recommendations

- Trust your intuition! It is *your* body and *your* baby.
- Make up a carefully considered birth plan well ahead of labor and delivery, then be as ready as you can to alter it if necessary, due to unforeseen circumstances.
- Gather together your perfect birth team to support you in every way possible during this challenging and exhilarating experience. Choose professionals whom you trust to be thoroughly experienced, competent, and loving; and caring loved ones who can stay calm during an emergency. Don't forget to ask someone to videotape the birth if you wish to have a visual memento of your remarkable experience.
- Perhaps the most important advice to cope with labor is "Breathe, breathe, breathe."
- Change positions as needed to remain as comfortable as possible and keep the labor moving along.
- Create a birth setting with all of the elements that are most conducive to your well-being and to ushering into the world your newborn treasure.

- If you choose to use homeopathy during your labor, have all the potential medicines available, as well as access to an experienced homeopath if the need arises.
- In a pinch, if you want additional help and no homeopathic medicine fits your symptom picture, take five drops of Rescue Remedy under your tongue up to every half hour.
- Pace yourself. Rest, sleep, relax, take a gentle walk, ask for a massage—whatever is necessary to keep you focused or distracted as needed.
- Rely on your birth team to provide you with whatever you want and need to eat and drink. Remember to drink plenty of fluids to avoid dehydration.
- Take one step and make one decision at a time, depending on how the events unfold.
- If you need conventional medications, ask for them. If you have a strong preference to use them only if absolutely necessary, share this with your birth team members so they can encourage you to use other options and leave medication as a last resort.
- Don't try to do it all by yourself! This is a time for you to receive all the help you need in every way!

	Key Symptoms	Mind	Body	Worse	Better	Food & Drink
Aconite (Monkshood)	Ailments from fright or shock	Panic attacks	Great restlessness and fear of death during labor	Fright	Rest	Intense desire for cold drinks
	Extreme anxiety	Fear of being in a crowd	Os is tender and slow to dilate	Chill	Sweating	Crave beer and bitter drinks
	Fear that you will not survive childbirth	Claustrophobia	Vagina is hot and dry			
	Tremendous restlessness	Agoraphobia	You can't sleep after the delivery			
		You must have others around				
Caulophyllum (Blue cohosh)	Erratic pains all over the body	Excitable	Rigid os	Cold	Keeping warm	Worse from coffee
	Labor is stalled	Worried, apprehensive	Your uterus lacks muscle tone			
	Drawing, cramping, and shooting pains	Irritable	Pricking, needlelike pains in your cervix			
	Sore or stiff neck		Weak or irregular labor pains			
			False labor			
China (Peruvian bark)	Weakness from loss of body fluids	Daydreaming	Extreme exhaustion and weakness after labor	Loss of fluids	Hard pressure	Desire for cherries
	Periodic symptoms	You feel that others are picking on you	You can't bear to be touched during labor	Touch	Loosening clothes	
	Anemia	You fantasize about being a superheroine	Oversensitive to noise during labor	Being jarred		
	Your face is pale	Great appreciation of beauty				
Cimicifuga (Black cohosh)	Cramping pains	Gloomy, as if enveloped in a black cloud	Labor pains that bring on fainting	Labor	Wrapping up	Worse from alcohol
	Feel you are trapped	Feel that you are going crazy	Pains across the abdomen, from side to side	Drafts	Holding on to your thighs	Desire for cold water
	Nape of your neck is very sensitive to drafts	Sighing	Soreness and stiffness of the whole body after labor			
	Muscle soreness	Talkative; jump from one topic to another	Shiver during the first stage of labor			

Remedy						
Gelsemium (Yellow jasmine)	Dizzy, drowsy, droopy, and dull Wiped-out feeling Fear of speaking in public Pains begin in front and extend up the back, to the sides, and down limbs	**Lack of courage** **Everything seems like an ordeal** **Feel you can't cope and must give up** **Want to be held so you don't shake**	**Loss of muscular power** **Sleepy and exhausted during labor** **Your labor makes no progress even though your os is fully dilated** Severe, sharp labor pains extending from uterus to back and hips	Fright Shock Surprise	Shaking Profuse urination	Better from alcohol Feel either better or worse from alcohol
Pulsatilla (Windflower)	Symptoms and moods change rapidly You cry very easily Hate being overheated Prefer being outside in the fresh air	**Soft, tender, sensitive** **You love being nurtured and can feel needy** **Very emotional** **Change your mind a lot**	**Urge to bend forward during labor pains** **Labor pains are slow, weak, and don't lead anywhere** Irregular, spasmodic labor pains that may lead to fainting Retained placenta	Heat Rich foods	**Being outside in the open air** **Walking slowly** Cold applications, food, or drink	**Crave rich foods, but they make you sick** **Not at all thirsty**
Sepia (Cuttlefish ink)	No interest in making love You feel turned off by your partner Worn out Love dancing and vigorous exercise	**Snappy and short with others** **Cry easily without wanting to** **No real interest in your family** **Want to be left alone**	**Delayed labor with weak labor pains** **Uterus feels heavy and dragging as if it would fall out** **No labor pains even though your os is dilated** **Constipated** Herpes during labor	Vinegar 4:00 to 6:00 P.M. Cold	**Vigorous exercise or dancing** **Keeping busy** Staying warm	**Craving for pickles and vinegar**

Mastitis (See also Breastfeeding Problems)

Description

Mastitis is an inflammation of the breast, usually occurring in nursing moms. It may be associated with a bacterial infection such as *Staphylococcus aureus,* but the discharge may also be sterile. Nursing, too, can frequently, in some women, lead to sore breasts and cracked nipples.

Symptoms

Mastitis is acutely painful, with swelling, engorgement, and inflammation of the breast tissue. Nursing, as well as expressing your breast milk, can be extremely uncomfortable.

Complications

Mastitis is usually a local problem, but a systemic infection can occur in rare cases. It is also possible to transmit infection to your nursing baby, requiring medical attention.

Look

Is your breast red or hot?
Is it tender to the touch?
What does your nipple look like?
Do you notice any discharge from your nipple? If so, what does it look or smell like?
Do you have a fever?

Listen

"Suddenly my breast got beet-red and swollen and I got a fever."
    Belladonna
"Any time I move, even a little, my breast hurts." *Bryonia*
"My nipples are very dry, cracked, and sore." *Castor equi*
"My breasts hurt in between nursing and the pain goes all the way to my back." *Phellandrium*
"My lymph nodes are swollen and my breast pain radiates throughout my whole body." *Phytolacca*
"I feel exhausted and I can't sleep because my breast burns." *Silica*

Ask

How does you breast feel?

What makes the discomfort or pain better or worse?

How does nursing your baby affect your symptoms?

Have you been through any particular emotional traumas or changes lately?

Are you unusually hungry or thirsty? For what?

Do you feel particularly warm or chilly?

Pointers for Finding Your Homeopathic Medicine

• Mastitis that comes on suddenly with a high fever, red face and breast, and is worse on the right side indicates *Belladonna.*

• If your breast pain is much worse from any movement and you are cranky, think of *Bryonia.*

• If your breast pain occurs even from going down stairs and your nipples are sore and cracked, *Castor equi* is a strong possibility.

• If your nipples are very cracked and sore to the touch, consider *Castor equi* first, then *Phytolacca,* especially if you have any glandular swelling.

• *Hepar sulphuris* is useful if you feel chilly, sensitive, and touchy and experience splinterlike pains and have a foul, cheesy discharge from your breast.

• For breast pain that radiates to your back and is unbearable between nursing, take *Phellandrium.*

• For swollen lymph nodes in the armpit, use *Phytolacca* if your pain radiates to your entire body, and *Silica* if you have burning pains in the breast at night.

Dosage

• Take three pellets of 30C every four hours until you see an improvement.

• If you are no better after three doses, change medicines.

• After you first notice you have improved, take another dose only if your symptoms begin to return.

• Lower potencies (6X, 6C, and 30X) may need to be given more often (every one to two hours, depending on the severity of the mastitis).

• Higher potencies (200X, 200C, and 1M) usually need to be taken only once but may need a repetition if the symptoms are severe or return after initial improvement.

What to Expect

Mastitis should improve after taking homeopathic medicines within twenty-four to forty-eight hours. If successful, homeopathy will allow you to avoid antibiotics, which can complicate the problem by causing secondary yeast infections of your nipple and of your baby's oral mucous membranes.

Women's Naturopathic Self-Care Recommendations

• Alternating hot (five minutes) and cold (one minute) wet compresses stimulates circulation and healing.

• Specific massage techniques that promote drainage of the lymph system can help.

• Take an *Echinacea* and goldenseal combination: two dropperfuls of tincture in water three times a day, or six capsules a day, to stimulate your immune system. Discontinue if it affects you or the baby negatively or does not help within three days.

• Take beta-carotene (50,000 IU once a day).

• Take zinc (30 mg once a day).

• Take vitamin C (1,000 mg three times a day).

• If you have any persistent problems with nursing that lead you to consider weaning your baby early, call your local La Leche League. They can provide a wealth of practical information.

	Key Symptoms	Mind	Body	Worse	Better	Food & Drink
Belladonna (Deadly nightshade)	Mastitis comes on suddenly and violently Mastitis is often right-sided Breast is heavy, hard, inflamed, and red	Irritable Intense Vivacious Exuberant	**Throbbing breast pain** Streaks radiate from nipples	Jarring Lying down 3:00 P.M.	Sitting up in a quiet, dark room	Not usually thirsty Desire for lemons or lemonade, sour food, and cold water
Bryonia (Wild hops)	Breast pain worse from any motion Must hold the breasts when going up or down stairs Breasts are heavy, painful, and stony hard, but not very red	Want to go home Extremely irritable Keep thinking about business	**Inflamed breasts with suppressed flow of milk** Swollen left breast, hurts when lifting arm Nipples very hard Pain from motion of chest	Touch Deep breathing Coughing	Pressure Lying on the painful side	Thirst for large quantities of cold water Desire for coffee, wine, and acidic drinks
Castor equi (Rudimentary thumbnail of the horse)	Sore, deeply cracked nipples in nursing mothers Clothing touching the nipples is unbearable Dry, painful nipples with red around the areola Ulcerated nipples	Laughing at serious things or for no reason Dream of sick people	**Breast abscess** **Violent itching of the breast** **Pain in the breast after the birth** Breasts are swollen and tender, feeling as if they would fall off when going down stairs Breasts feel better from firm pressure	After childbirth Nursing	No pressure or touch	Desire for bread and tobacco
Hepar sulphuris (Calcium sulfide)	Breast is very painful, especially to touch Splinterlike pains in the breast Extreme sensitivity to cold air and applications	Extremely irritable and touchy Very sensitive to pain	**Breast abscess with thick pus** **Discharge from the breast smells sour or like rotten cheese** Swollen lymph glands under the armpit	Touch Lying on the painful part Drafts Uncovering	Warmth Covering up	Desire for vinegar Aversion to fats

continued on next page

127

	Key Symptoms	Mind	Body	Worse	Better	Food & Drink
Phellandrium (Water dropwort)	**Unbearable pain between nursing** **Pain in the nipples while nursing the child** **Pain in the right breast extending to the back between the shoulder blades**	Anxious about your health Fear that someone is behind you	**Pain in the breasts during the menstrual period** **Pain in the breasts which goes to the abdomen**	Breathing Cold air	Motion Open air	Desire for sour milk, beer Aversion to water
Phytolacca (Poke-root)	**Breasts heavy, stony hard, swollen, and tender** **Extreme pain in the breasts while nursing, worse in the left breast** **Breast pain radiates to the whole body**	Very afraid that you will die Don't care if you expose your body to others	**Sore all over** **Swollen lymph nodes in the arm pit** **Nipples are cracked, sensitive, and can be inverted**	Motion Lifting the breast	Lying on abdomen or left side Rest	Hunger soon after eating
Silica (Flint)	**Breast swollen, dark red, sensitive** **Burning pains prevent sleep** **Inflamed breast with a high fever**	Refined Delicate features	**Inflammation of nipples** **Darting, burning pain in left nipple** **Breast abscess** **Swollen lymph nodes in the armpit** **Low stamina and energy**	Warmth and heat	Cold, dampness Touch	Desire for eggs and sweets Aversion to fat and milk

Menstrual Pain *(Acute)*

Description

Menstrual cramping is pain of any kind associated with your period. It generally occurs during your flow but may occur before or after your period or at ovulation.

Symptoms

Mild to severe, or even debilitating pain of your ovaries, uterus, pelvic area, or pubic area, may be accompanied by back pain or general body discomfort. Pain may also radiate to your thighs. Along with cramps, you may also experience headaches, nausea, diarrhea, or constipation, as well as a variety of mental and emotional symptoms such as mood swings, depression, anxiety, and irritability.

Complications

Recurrent menstrual pain may sometimes be an indication of a more serious problem, such as endometriosis, ovarian cysts, uterine fibroids, or rarely, cancer.

Look

Is your coloring or facial expression out of the ordinary?
Are you visibly in pain or discomfort?
Does being in any special position make you feel better or worse?

Listen

"My right ovary is throbbing terribly and I'm ticked off." *Belladonna*
"It feels like there's a tight band around my abdomen and it's driving me up a wall!" *Cactus grandifolia*
"No, nothing makes me feel any better. Just get out of my sight before I throw something!" *Chamomilla*
"All I want to do is lie down and curl up in a little ball." *Colocynthis*
"I need a heating pad on my uterus." *Magnesia phosphorica*
"My cramps are worse after I drink too much wine before my period."
  Nux vomica

Ask

How do I feel?

What bothers me the most about my periods?

Where am I in my cycle?

Have I gone through this before?

Am I in pain? If so, where exactly is it?

Does my pain stay in one place or does it radiate elsewhere? If so, where?

How intense is the pain?

What makes it better or worse?

Have I experienced any other symptoms?

Do I have any mental or emotional symptoms along with my cramps?

Pointers for Finding Your Homeopathic Medicine

- If you have heavy, bright-red bleeding, gushing, and throbbing pain, *Belladonna* is a good bet.
- If the pain is better from heat and pressure, think first of *Magnesia phosphorica,* then of *Colocynthis.*
- For pain so violent that you feel like screaming, take *Cactus.*
- If your pain is very intense and you feel downright nasty, kind of like a kid throwing a tantrum, look at *Chamomilla.*
- If you feel better when you draw your knees up to your chest, consider *Colocynthis.*
- If your menstrual pain begins just after an episode of anger, you may need *Nux vomica* or, if it doesn't help, *Colocynthis* or *Bryonia.*
- If your cramps came on directly after drinking too much alcohol or overeating rich foods, try *Nux vomica.*

Dosage

- Take three pellets of 30C every three to four hours until you see an improvement.
- If you are no better after three doses, change medicines.
- After you first notice you have improved, take another dose only if your symptoms begin to return.
- Lower potencies (6X, 6C, and 30X) may need to be given more often (every one to two hours, depending on the severity of the symptoms).
- Higher potencies (200X, 200C, and 1M) usually need to be taken only once but may need a repetition if the symptoms are severe or return after initial improvement.

What to Expect

Homeopathic medicines generally help to relieve pain within five minutes to several hours, though it may take longer. Self-treatment for menstrual pain can be very effective, but if the symptoms recur each month, are severe, and do not respond to your own treatment, do consult an experienced homeopathic practitioner for help.

Women's Naturopathic Self-Care Recommendations

• Take a sitz bath. Fill the tub with hot water up to two inches below your navel. Sit with your knees bent. Stay in the tub for five minutes. Then squat in a tub of cold water for one minute. Repeat the cycle two to three times. Walking, stretching, and other physical exercise can often reduce pain and discomfort.

• Massage of your pressure points can promote circulation of blood flow and energy and decrease discomfort.

• For muscle cramps, calcium (1,000 mg) and magnesium (500 mg) can help.

• Take *Viburnum* (cramp bark) tincture: one-half teaspoon every hour, up to six doses, or one capsule three to four times a day.

• A heating pad is often useful.

• Castor packs to the abdomen, applied along with a heating pad, can relieve pain.

• Avoid caffeine and salt premenstrually.

• Certain foods, such as beef, pork, lamb, poultry, and dairy products, may aggravate prostaglandin production and exacerbate uterine cramps. Fish oil (1,000 mg EPA and 700 mg DHA) or evening primrose oil (500 mg, three times a day) enhance prostaglandin secretion.

• Do not smoke.

• Tampons and IUDs may aggravate menstrual pain.

	Key Symptoms	Mind	Body	Worse	Better	Food & Drink
Belladonna *(Deadly nightshade)*	**Throbbing pains, worse on the right side** **Sudden onset of symptoms** **Violent pain** **Feeling of fullness in the uterus from congested blood** **Right-sided symptoms**	Irritable Maddening pain	**Profuse, bright red, gushing, clotted menstrual flow** **Bearing down sensation, as if the pelvic organs would fall out**	**Motion** Light Noise	Semi-erect position Lying in bed Leaning against something	**Great thirst for cold water, or no thirst at all** Desire for lemons and lemonade
Cactus grandifolia *(Night-blooming cereus)*	**Extreme pain that feels like a band across the abdomen** **Violent menstrual pains** **Screams with menstrual pain**	Cry without knowing why Don't think you'll ever feel better	**Clotted menstrual flow with pain as each clot is passed** Throbbing pain in the ovary Lumpy menstrual flow	Lying on the left side Exertion Walking	Being outside	Aversion to meat
Chamomilla *(Chamomile)*	**Intense, laborlike pain with the menstrual flow** **Profuse, dark, clotted blood with occasional gushing of bright red blood** **Menstrual pain after anger** **Hypersensitivity to pain** **Inconsolable**	**Very irritable** **Say you want something, then change your mind when you get it**	**Severe menstrual pain, with pains extending down the inner thighs** Greenish diarrhea	Lying in bed	**Being rocked** Cold applications	Thirsty for cold drinks
Colocynthis *(Bitter cucumber)*	**Cramping pain that is relieved by bending over double** **Menstrual pain made more tolerable by hard pressure** **Symptoms after anger**	Irritable and indignant Feelings hurt easily	**Pain so intense that you vomit** Menstrual pain relieved by heat and pressure Ovarian pain	**Anger** **Lying on the painless side**	After a bowel movement or passing gas Heat	Very thirsty Aggravation from starchy food

Magnesia phosphorica (*Magnesium phosphate*)	Pain relieved by heat and pressure Menstrual pain before the period Pain feels better when the menstrual flow begins Menstrual flow is dark and too early	Irritable Want nurturing, feel like you were not nurtured as a child	Great weakness with the menstrual period Intense soreness and bruised feeling in the abdomen Ovarian pain Swelling of the labia	Lying on the right side Drafts	**Hot baths** **Bending**	Milk aggravates Thirst for very cold drinks
Nux vomica (*Quaker's button*)	**Cramps extend to the whole body** **Menstrual pain with the urge for a bowel movement** **Menstrual cramping after anger, rich foods, or too much alcohol**	**Irritable and impatient** **Obsessed with business** **Competitive and hard-driving, Type A** Easily offended	Menstrual flow is profuse, early, and lasts too long Heavy bleeding after too much coffee, alcohol, rich foods	Pressure Tight clothing around waist	Rest Lying on either side	**Desire for fats, spicy food, alcohol, and stimulants**

Miscarriage

Description

A miscarriage, also known as a spontaneous abortion, is the loss of the fetus before the twentieth week of pregnancy. Approximately 20 to 30 percent of women have cramping or bleeding at some time during this period and 10 to 15 percent suffer a miscarriage. It is thought that a high percentage of miscarriages are due to abnormalities in the fetus. Women who miscarry tend to lose their babies most often between the eighth and twelfth week after conception. Causes include an incompetent cervix, hormonal imbalances, abnormalities of the uterus, hypothyroidism, diabetes, acute infections, crack use, severe emotional shock, and viruses.

Symptoms

The primary symptoms are cramping and bleeding. Pain tends to be more severe the longer the pregnancy has progressed and can, when extreme, resemble labor pains. Miscarriage is confirmed by pelvic ultrasound, which shows the absence of a fetal heartbeat.

Complications

The main complication is infection, or septic abortion, and is characterized by chills, fever, and if extreme, shock.

Look

Has my facial expression or appearance changed?

Have I experienced any uterine bleeding? If so, what is the color and quantity?

Do I notice myself favoring any particular position?

Listen

"I have this awful premonition that I won't survive giving birth." *Aconite*

"My right ovary stings and burns." *Apis*

"I have such pain in my back and pubis and I feel really weak." *Caulophyllum*

"Ever since I started to bleed, I feel completely wrung out." *China*

"Losing my baby has completely devastated me. I can't go on." *Ignatia*

"Please don't leave me. I'm afraid I'll miscarry and I just can't be alone."
   Pulsatilla
"My blood flow is bright red and profuse, and the clots are dark red."
   Sabina
"My uterus feels so heavy. Like it will just fall through the floor." *Sepia*

Ask

Did anything happen just before I began to miscarry?

What are my specific symptoms?

What bothers me the most?

Am I in pain? How much?

If I'm bleeding, how much?

How is my energy?

Do I have chills or a fever?

How do I feel mentally and emotionally?

What makes me feel better or worse?

Can I handle this myself or do I need professional help?

Pointers for Finding Your Homeopathic Medicine

• For threatened miscarriages resulting from fear, take *Aconite* immediately.

• If the main symptom is stinging ovarian pain and you have lost your thirst, consider *Apis mellifica*.

• If you feel weak and your uterus is unresponsive, *Caulophyllum* is likely to help.

• *China* is the best medicine for weakness after bleeding.

• If grief and sadness, expressed by either sobbing or silence, is predominant, think of *Ignatia*.

• *Pulsatilla* is the medicine of choice for soft, sensitive, changeable, affectionate women in danger of having a miscarriage.

• The key symptom for *Sabina* is pain extending from the pelvis to the pubis.

• *Sepia* is the first medicine to consider for a woman who is miscarrying and wants nothing to do with her partner.

Dosage

• Take three pellets of 30C every half-hour to four hours, depending on your symptoms, until you see an improvement.

- If you are no better after three doses, change medicines.
- After you first notice you have improved, take another dose only if your symptoms begin to return.
- Lower potencies (6X, 6C, and 30X) may need to be given more often (every one to two hours, depending on the severity of the symptoms).
- Higher potencies (200X, 200C, and 1M) usually need to be taken only once but may need a repetition if the symptoms are severe or return after initial improvement.

What to Expect

You should feel better within fifteen minutes to three days after taking the correct medicine depending on the intensity of your symptoms. Unless you are very comfortable treating yourself during a miscarriage without medical attention or have suffered a number of miscarriages and know what to expect, it is advisable to consult with your obstetrician or midwife.

Women's Naturopathic Self-Care Recommendations

- If you feel that you are in danger of miscarrying, take it easy and avoid lifting anything heavy.
- In most cases, it is advisable to go along with your daily routine, avoiding vigorous activities. Some women, especially those with repeated miscarriages, may need bed rest to maintain their pregnancies.
- Drink plenty of fluids.
- Avoid hot, spicy food; alcohol; and caffeine.
- No smoking or drugs of any kind are allowed during pregnancy.
- Relax, pray, and be good to yourself.
- If you do start to miscarry, remind yourself that it is a common, though traumatic, event, and don't blame yourself for anything you might have done differently.
- Massaging pressure points can be very helpful in decreasing pain.
- If your miscarriage is early and the pain is not severe, you can probably handle it on your own. If the pain is severe, you are uncertain whether the fetus is still alive, or you need pain medication, consult your obstetrician or midwife. Dilation and curettage (D & C) may not be required.
- If you miscarry, allow yourself and your partner to experience the emotional, as well as physical, pain and grief. You may choose to hold a ritual in honor of the child you lost.

	Key Symptoms	Mind	Body	Worse	Better	Food & Drink
Aconite *(Monkshood)*	You become sick after a fearful event, recent or past Fear you will die during childbirth Miscarriage from fright, excitement, or anger Dizziness or fainting, being really scared	Anxiety, with great excitability and nervousness You feel beside yourself Panic attacks Fear of crowds	Violent labor pains Rapid breathing and pulse Great restlessness Bleeding from the uterus	Fright Chill	Rest Sweating	Intense desire for cold drinks You crave beer and bitter drinks
Apis mellifica *(Honeybee)*	Burning, stinging pain Swelling Affected area is hot and red Inflammations	Busy Jealous Protective of your home and family Hard to please	Miscarriage in your second to fourth month Profuse bleeding with your miscarriage Stinging pain in one or both ovaries preceding labor pains Little urination or thirst	Heat, hot rooms, hot bath	Cool air, cold applications, cold bath or shower	Lack of thirst
Caulophyllum *(Blue cohosh)*	Uterine problems Pains dart from place to place Drawing, cramping, and shooting pains Sore or stiff neck	Weak, nervous Apprehensive Excitable Easily dissatisfied	Repeated miscarriages due to weakness of the uterus Miscarriage with little or no flooding Severe pain in back and pubic region Tormenting, irregular contractions	Cold	Warmth	Worse from coffee
China *(Peruvian bark)*	Hemorrhages Weakness after loss of blood or other bodily fluids Symptoms occur intermittently Gas and bloating	You fantasize about doing great things Think others intentionally pick on you You can't seem to act on your ideas and visions	Weakness since the miscarriage Hemorrhage after miscarriage Tremendous abdominal bloating not relieved by passing gas	Loss of fluids Touch Being jarred	Hard pressure Loosening clothes	Desire for cherries

continued on next page

	Key Symptoms	Mind	Body	Worse	Better	Food & Drink
Ignatia (St. Ignatius bean)	Grief or loss Uncontrollable crying Frequent sighing Unpredictable mood swings and symptoms	Uncontrollable sobbing You feel devastated High-strung Extremely sensitive and emotional	Miscarriage from grief Recurrent tendency to miscarry Miscarriage from suppressed grief Loss of appetite	Grief, loss, disappointment	Deep breathing Changing positions	Strong like or dislike of fruit Desire for cheese
Pulsatilla (Windflower)	One of the best medicines for hormonal problems Symptoms are very changeable You are soft, warm, nurturing, and want to be loved You can't stand a warm room with windows closed	Your moods change rapidly You cry easily Hate being overheated Prefer being outside	Bleeding stops, then returns with twice the intensity Pains and bleeding alternate Flow of blood occurs every now and then during pregnancy Miscarriage in early months of pregnancy Fainting spells	Heat Rich food	Being outside in the open air Walking slowly Cold applications, food, or drink	You crave rich foods, but they make you sick Not at all thirsty
Sabina (Savine)	Uterine problems One of the best homeopathic medicines for miscarriage Women's problems after miscarriage Uterine bleeding with bright-red blood and dark clots	Highly irritable and anxious Extreme sensitivity to music Sensitive to noise Depressed	Threatened miscarriage, especially in the third month Drawing pain in the small of the back, penetrating right through your pelvis to your pubis Blood is bright red, thin, and liquid or has dark red clots Blood comes out in gushes and is more profuse on movement	Heat You can't stand to hear music Night	Cold	Crave sour, juicy, refreshing things
Sepia (Cuttlefish ink)	You have no desire to make love You feel turned off toward your partner Worn out Love dancing and vigorous exercise	You feel very depressed about your threatened miscarriage You feel indifferent toward your loved ones You want to be left alone Cranky and weepy	Repeated miscarriages Bearing down or dragging sensation as if your uterus will fall out Severe itching of your vulva Tendency to miscarry in the fifth to seventh month Retained placenta after miscarriage	Vinegar 4:00 to 6:00 P.M. Cold	Vigorous exercise or dancing Keeping busy Staying warm	You crave pickles and vinegar

Morning Sickness

Description

Morning sickness occurs most commonly during your first three months of pregnancy but may persist, in some cases, throughout the entire pregnancy. Although it is called "morning sickness," the symptoms are by no means confined to the early hours of the day.

Symptoms

Nausea, mild to awful, are most characteristic, and you may also vomit. You may have a tremendous aversion to the sight, smell, or even the idea of eating food.

Complications

Apart from the discomfort and inconvenience, the main complication of prolonged morning sickness is malnutrition and your inability gain appropriate weight, possibly resulting in a low birth weight or congenital health problems for your baby. But, despite even extreme morning sickness, your baby is likely to be fine even if you just want to die from nausea. Hyperemesis gravidarum—intense, uncontrollable vomiting during pregnancy, often associated with liver disease—is a much more severe complication and may cause dehydration and acidosis, necessitating hospitalization and intravenous fluids.

Look

Is my face pale?

Do I notice any other visible changes in myself since I developed morning sickness?

Do I vomit? If so, how often?

Do I prefer to be in a particular posture or position to be more comfortable?

Listen

"My nausea has been much worse since I was up all last night taking care of my two-year-old daughter." *Cocculus*

"The nausea is even worse when I ride in the car (boat, airplane)." *Cocculus, Sepia, Tabacum*

"The sight or smell of food absolutely nauseates me." *Cocculus, Colchicum, Ipecac, Sepia*

"My nausea is constant and even vomiting doesn't help." *Ipecac*

"I want to vomit but I can't." *Kreosotum*

"No sex for me." *Sepia*

"I feel green, almost like when I tried that first cigarette as a teenager." *Tabacum*

"I break out in a cold sweat with the morning sickness. All I want is something icy." *Veratrum*

Ask

How long have I been pregnant?

How long have I felt nauseous and/or been vomiting?

What are my symptoms and how severe are they?

What brings on my nausea?

Is it worse at any specific time of the day or night?

Does anything make my nausea/vomiting better or worse?

Am I hungry or thirsty?

Do I crave any particular food or drink?

Is there any food or drink I just can't tolerate?

Can I keep anything down?

Are there any other symptoms?

Pointers for Finding Your Homeopathic Medicine

• The most common medicines for morning sickness are *Sepia* and *Colchicum.*

• When aversion to the smell of food is the strongest symptom, consider *Colchicum* first.

• For severe vomiting, use *Ipecac,* and for the most terrible nausea, use *Tabacum.*

• When aversion to sex is a strong symptom, consider *Sepia* or *Kreosotum.*

• *Sepia* is for conditions that are much better from vigorous exercise or dancing, which differentiates it from the motion sickness medicines such as *Tabacum* and *Cocculus.* The latter two are for symptoms that are much worse, not better, from motion.

• *Veratrum* is the medicine of choice if you are very cold, suffer from vomiting and diarrhea, and would die for fruit, ice, and sour foods like pickles or lemons.

Dosage

- Take three pellets of 30C twice a day until you see an improvement.
- If you are no better after three doses, change medicines.
- After you first notice you have improved, take another dose only if your symptoms begin to return.
- Lower potencies (6X, 6C, and 30X) may need to be given more often (every one to two hours, depending on the severity of the nausea).
- Higher potencies (200X, 200C, and 1M) usually need to be taken only once but may need a repetition if the symptoms are severe or return after initial improvement.

What to Expect

Homeopathic medicines are very safe to use during pregnancy. The symptoms are generally relieved within several days to a week or ten days. Even though homeopathy is very safe, it is best not to take too many homeopathic medicines during pregnancy. If you have tried two or three without success or if your morning sickness lasts past the third month of pregnancy, consult a homeopath for constitutional treatment.

Women's Naturopathic Self-Care Recommendations

- Eat small amounts of food frequently.
- Grab a bite before getting up in the morning.
- Chew Saltine crackers to help relieve the nausea.
- Stick to bland foods such as broth, rice, and pasta.
- Tea (preferably herbal) and toast are usually well-tolerated.
- Sipping ginger root tea is a time-tested reliever of nausea. Use a one-quarter-inch slice of ginger root boiled in a cup of water for fifteen minutes.
- Many herbs, such as pennyroyal, need to be avoided during pregnancy. Research carefully before using any herbs, especially in your first trimester. Stimulating Stomach 36, an acupressure point in the soft place between the knee and to the outside of the leg where the tibia and fibula bones meet, often helps to alleviate nausea. Use firm rotary pressure on the spot for several seconds. Repeat as needed.

	Key Symptoms	Mind	Body	Worse	Better	Food & Drink
Cocculus (Indian cockle)	Nausea from the sight or smell of food Any kind of motion sickness with vertigo Nausea from looking at moving objects or watching things out of the window of a moving vehicle	**Anxiety about the welfare of loved ones** Do not like to be interrupted or disturbed	**Must lie down with the morning sickness, or gets nauseated** Headache, nausea, and vomiting with the morning sickness	**Loss of sleep** **Taking care of a loved one who is ill** Emotional stress Open air	Lying on your side	Aversion to food
Colchicum (Meadow saffron)	Intolerance of smells, especially cooking food Nausea from the smell of cooked meat, fish, and eggs Symptoms made worse by motion and turning the head Severe vomiting and retching	Ailments in response to rudeness of others Anger at trifles	Hungry, but disgusted at the thought of eating or when you smell food Vomit is stringy and clear Swallowing saliva induces vomiting	Eggs Change of weather Cold, dampness	Warmth Rest	Detest sight or smell of food, especially fish, eggs, and soup Eggs disagree
Ipecac (Ipecac root)	Terrible, constant nausea, not relieved by vomiting Nausea and vomiting with nearly all conditions Nausea with a clean tongue Hate food and the smell of food	Difficult to please Don't know what you want	**Bleeding and nausea at the same time** Cramps in the abdomen Drooling with the nausea	**Vomiting** **Warmth** Overeating	Open air	**Not thirsty** Desire for sweets, pastries
Kreosotum (Creosote)	Nausea with desire to vomit, but can't Continuous vomiting with lots of straining Vomits sweetish water, undigested food, and everything that is eaten	Dissatisfied with everything Afraid when thinking about having sex	Vomit lots of sour, acrid fluid or foamy, white mucus Drooling during pregnancy Very irritating, burning, corrosive vaginal discharge	Cold Lying down	Warmth Hot food	**Desire for smoked food**

Remedy	Symptoms	Emotional	Stomach	Worse	Better	Desires/Aversions
Sepia (*Cuttlefish ink*)	**Sensitive to the thought or smell of food, even her favorites** / **Motion sickness from walking or riding in the car** / **Stomach feels empty, but eating doesn't help** / **The smell of food cooking makes you nauseated**	**Aversion to your partner and sex** / Irritable / Depressed and crying	Crosses your legs to keep the uterus from falling out / Threatened miscarriage	**Vinegar** / **Afternoon** / Too much sex / Fasting or missing a meal / Cold	Exercise, dancing / **Keeping busy** / Warmth	**Desire for vinegar, sour food, sweets** / Aversion to fat, salt
Tabacum (*Tobacco*)	**Deathly nauseous** / **Cold, clammy, and pale with the nausea** / **Motion sickness, seasickness from the least motion** / **Better from cold fresh air** / **Spitting with the nausea**	Feel confused, wretched	**Violent vomiting from the least motion** / Profuse sweat and saliva / Sinking feeling in the stomach	**Heat** / **Opening the eyes**	Uncovering the abdomen / Fresh air / Cold applications	Crave tobacco
Veratrum album (*White hellebore*)	**Violent vomiting and diarrhea** / **Cold sweat on the forehead while vomiting** / **Icy cold, with cold sweat**	**Very active and busy** / **Restless**	**Projectile vomiting** / **Abdominal cramping** / Collapse with a bluish color / Diarrhea very forceful, followed by exhaustion and cold sweat	**Cold** / Cold drinks / Fruit	Warmth / Hot drinks / Covering up	**Desire for sour food, juicy fruit, pickles, lemons, salt, and ice**

Motion Sickness

Description

Motion sickness, also known as sea-, air-, or car-sickness, is a combination of symptoms caused by stimulation of the balance mechanism in the inner ear due to repeated motion. Disorientation, without being able to see a fixed horizon during motion, can induce motion sickness. Emotional stress can sometimes aggravate motion sickness.

Symptoms

Nausea and vomiting are the main symptoms. Salivation, sweating, paleness, and hyperventilation are also common. You may feel confused or disoriented as well.

Complications

Dehydration and lack of eating can produce problems if your motion sickness is prolonged.

Look

Am I flushed or pale?
Do I sweat more or less than usual?
How rapid is my pulse?
Do I favor any particular body position to try to feel better?

Listen

"Can't we please stop moving?" *Cocculus*
"If I could just get some sleep, I'm sure I would start to feel better."
    Cocculus
"I feel so confused that I don't know right from left. Could you please
    take me home?" *Petroleum*
"Whenever the ship heaves, I do too, unless I'm dancing." *Sepia*
"I feel so bad. Just like when I first started smoking." *Tabacum*

Ask

When did my motion sickness begin?
How bad do I feel?

What are my exact symptoms?

What brings on my nausea (and vomiting)?

Does anything make me feel better or worse?

Am I hungry or thirsty?

Does any food or drink appeal to me?

Is there anything I just can't stand eating or drinking?

Can I keep anything down?

Do I experience any pain or other symptoms along with the motion sickness?

How do I feel emotionally?

Pointers for Finding Your Homeopathic Medicine

- *Cocculus* is best when looking at passing objects makes you feel worse.
- *Petroleum* is particularly good for motion sickness with confusion and disorientation.
- For motion sickness relieved by vigorous exercise or dancing, choose *Sepia*.
- *Tabacum* is excellent for really severe motion sickness, in which you feel so bad, you just want to die.

Dosage

- Take three pellets of 30C every three to four hours until you see an improvement.
- If you are no better after three doses, change medicines.
- After you first notice you have improved, take another dose only if your symptoms begin to return.
- Lower potencies (6X, 6C, and 30X) may need to be given more often (every one to two hours, depending on the severity of the motion sickness).
- Higher potencies (200X, 200C, and 1M) usually need to be taken only once but may need a repetition if the symptoms are severe or return after initial improvement.

What to Expect

Homeopathic medicines can rapidly relieve motion sickness within minutes. If yours is prolonged or recurrent, you may want to consult a physician to rule out other problems or seek out constitutional homeopathic treatment.

Women's Naturopathic Self-Care Recommendations

- Try to sit in the place in the vehicle where there is the least motion.
- Stare at a fixed point, rather than at a moving object.
- Lying down or reclining may help.
- Look above the horizon at a forty-five-degree angle.
- Get some fresh air.
- Eat small amounts of food often.
- Saltine crackers may help relieve your nausea.
- Eat bland foods such as toast, broth, rice, and pasta if you have any appetite.
- Drink fluids to avoid dehydration.
- Ginger in the form of ginger ale or ginger root tea is often rapidly helpful. Use a one-quarter-inch slice of fresh ginger root boiled in a cup of water for fifteen minutes.
- Stimulate Stomach 36, an acupressure point in the soft place below the stomach and to the outside of the leg where the tibia and the fibula bones meet. Use firm rotary pressure on the spot for several seconds. Repeat as needed.

	Key Symptoms	Mind	Body	Worse	Better	Food & Drink
Cocculus (*Indian cockle*)	**Any kind of motion sickness** Nausea from looking at moving objects or watching things out of the window of a moving vehicle	Don't like to be interrupted or disturbed Nervous exhaustion, confusion, and disorientation	**Must lie down** Headache, nausea, and vomiting with morning sickness Nausea from the sight or smell of food	**Loss of sleep** **Caring for a loved one who is ill** Emotional stress Open air Touch	Lying on your side	**Aversion to food** Craving for beef
Petroleum (*Coal oil*)	**Seasickness, airsickness, or motion sickness** Sensation of great emptiness in the stomach relieved by constant eating	**Disoriented** Can't make up your mind Irritable	**Nausea from hunger** Heartburn Motion sickness with dry, cracked eczema	**Riding in a car, plane, or boat** Cold weather	Warm air Dry weather	**Desire for beer** Aversion to meat, fats, and cooked or hot foods
Sepia (*Cuttlefish ink*)	**Motion sickness from walking or riding in the car** Sensitivity to the thought or smell of food, even your favorites Nausea caused by the smell of cooking food	**Aversion to partner and to sex** Irritable Depressed and crying	**Stomach feels empty but eating doesn't help** Constipation	**Vinegar** Pregnancy Fasting or missing a meal Cold	**Vigorous exercise, dancing** Keeping busy Warmth	**Desire for vinegar,** sour food, sweets Aversion to fat, salt
Tabacum (*Tobacco*)	**Deathly nauseous** **Cold, clammy, and pale with the nausea** **Motion sickness, seasickness from the least motion** Symptoms relieved by cold fresh air Spitting with the nausea	Feel wretched Confusion	**Violent vomiting induced by the least motion** Profuse sweat and saliva Sinking feeling in the stomach	**Heat** **Opening your eyes**	Uncovering the abdomen Fresh air Cold applications	Crave tobacco

Performance Anxiety

PERFORMANCE ANXIETY

Description
Performance anxiety, also called stage fright, is nervousness or anxiety prior to a performance or presentation. It is said to be the number one fear of people in America.

Symptoms
You may feel weak, look pale, and have butterflies in your stomach, as well as experience shaking, trembling, diarrhea, rapid heartbeat and pulse, and perspiration.

Complications
There are no severe complications; however, fainting can occur.

Look
Do I have any visible symptoms of performance anxiety?
What is the color of my face?
Am I trembling? Perspiring?

Listen
"What if I forget all of my lines? What if I go blank? What if I faint?"
   Argentum nitricum
"I feel so shaky and dizzy. I'm really, really afraid." *Gelsemium*
"My worst fear is getting up in front of all of those people and making a
   fool of myself." *Lycopodium*
"If I can't do it perfectly, I might as well not do it at all." *Silica*

Ask
What am I feeling?
What are my physical symptoms?
What is my mental and emotional state?
When did these symptoms start?
What bothers me the most?
Have I had this before?
What makes me feel better or worse?

Pointers for Finding Your Homeopathic Medicine

• For extreme anxiety with rapid heartbeat and an irrational fear about what is about to occur, take *Argentum nitricum.*

• If there is weakness, trembling, dizziness, and diarrhea, consider *Gelsemium* first.

• If your main concern is the risk of making a fool of yourself, *Lycopodium* will probably help you.

• *Silica* is the best choice if you are proper, refined, and must do everything according to the acceptable standard.

Dosage

• Take three pellets of 30C one to two hours prior to the event or performance. Repeat every thirty minutes until there is improvement.

• After you first notice you have improved, take another dose only if your symptoms begin to return.

• Lower potencies (6X, 6C, and 30X) may need to be given more often (every one to two hours, depending on the severity of the performance anxiety).

• Higher potencies (200X, 200C, and 1M) usually need to be taken only once but may need a repetition if the symptoms are severe or return after initial improvement.

What to Expect

You should notice a definite improvement within five to thirty minutes.

Women's Naturopathic Self-Care Recommendations

• Count slowly from one to one hundred, taking long, deep breaths.

• Visualize or imagine your last successful performance or presentation.

• Think of everyone who is present as a friend who wants you to do your best.

• Sip a glass of room-temperature water.

• Splash cold water on your face.

• Tense and relax your muscles to release your nervousness.

• If homeopathic medicines are not available, take five drops of Rescue Remedy (a Bach Flower Essence) every fifteen to thirty minutes, beginning one to two hours prior to the event.

	Key Symptoms	Mind	Body	Worse	Better	Food & Drink
Argentum nitricum (Silver nitrate)	Anxiety in anticipation of an event Keep asking yourself, "What if this or that happens?" Fear of being late Wake in the morning feeling that you can't face the day	Anxiety in crowds, closed rooms, elevators, theaters, airplanes Hurried Impulsive Talk a lot	Violent palpitations that make you feel that your heart will jump out of your body Diarrhea from anticipation	Tight spaces Crowds Heat	Cool air	Strong desire for sweets, salt, and cheese
Gelsemium (Yellow jasmine)	Stage fright with trembling, chills, weakness, and dizziness Anxiety from anticipation Hoarseness or laryngitis from stage fright	Very frightened Confused and dazed	Tremendous fatigue Wiped out expression on her face Sticky perspiration all over the body Chills with trembling	Ordeals	Urination Alcoholic drinks	Lack of thirst
Lycopodium (Club moss)	Dread the presence of new people Fear of failure or of looking like a fool Loss of self-confidence from anticipation	Hate to undertake something new, but are usually okay once you begin Can be bossy Like appreciation and applause	Indigestion and diarrhea from fright Abdominal bloating and gas Full after eating small amounts of food	4:00 to 8:00 P.M. Warmth	Warm drinks	Strong desire for sweets and warm drinks
Silica (Flint)	Low stamina and energy Refined Must keep up your image You are polite and proper	You tend be mild and to give in Fastidious Shy in social settings and performances Feel that what you have to say is not important	Cold, clammy palms Profuse, sometimes bad-smelling, perspiration, especially feet Constipation Thin frame	Societal pressure Suppressed perspiration Cold	Wrapping up	Desire for eggs and sweets Aversion to fat and milk

150

PMS *(Mild)* (See also Fibrocystic Breasts)

Description

Premenstrual syndrome, also known as premenstrual tension, is a combination of physical, mental, and emotional symptoms ranging from mild to severe. PMS may begin from three days to two weeks before your period and it ends either when you start to bleed or within the first couple of days.

Symptoms

Physical symptoms are variable and extensive and may include fatigue; insomnia; breast pain; pelvic pain or discomfort; water retention and weight gain; back pain; gastrointestinal symptoms such as constipation, diarrhea, nausea, and bloating; and headaches. You may also experience mental and emotional complaints such as fogginess and confusion, anger, mood swings, depression, and anxiety. Any symptom that you normally have may get worse before your period.

Complications

Premenstrual anger can, in rare cases, lead to suicidal or homicidal rage.

Look

Has my appearance changed at all?
Do I favor a particular position?
Am I doing things that are out of character for me?

Listen

"My PMS has been terrible since I stopped taking the pill." *Folliculinum*
"My vaginal discharge burns so badly that I can't stand it." *Kreosotum*
"I just want to explode before my period." *Lachesis*
"My partner says I'm oversexed." *Lilium tigrinum*
"I just want to cry." *Pulsatilla*
"If my partner wants sex before my period, watch out!" *Sepia*

Ask

How do I feel overall?
Which physical symptom bothers me the most?
What makes it better or worse?

How is my thinking?
My energy?
My sexual desire?
What troubles me the most, emotionally?

Pointers for Finding Your Homeopathic Medicine

• If you have a variety of PMS symptoms that don't fit the other medicines listed here, particularly if you have used birth control pills, consider *Folliculinum*.

• *Kreosotum* is an excellent medicine for irritability along with an acrid vaginal discharge.

• *Lachesis* is the most common medicine for premenstrual anger that is relieved as soon as the period comes.

• If you are steaming mad but really want to make love, *Lilium tigrinum* is a good bet.

• *Pulsatilla* can be of great benefit if you feel ultrasensitive, weepy, and needy before your period.

• If your sexual energy evaporates before your period and you just want to be left alone, *Sepia* is likely to help.

Dosage

• Take three pellets of 30C every three to four hours until you see an improvement.

• If you are no better after three doses, change medicines.

• After you first notice you have improved, take another dose only if your symptoms begin to return.

• Lower potencies (6X, 6C, and 30X) may need to be given more often (every one to two hours, depending on the severity of your PMS).

• Higher potencies (200X, 200C, and 1M) usually need to be taken only once but may need a repetition if the symptoms are severe or return after initial improvement.

What to Expect

You should feel better within one to four days after taking the correct medicine. If your PMS occurs each month, is severe, or does not get better after trying a couple of the indicated homeopathic medicines, consult a homeopath, because PMS is part of your constitutional picture.

Women's Naturopathic Self-Care Recommendations

- Eat a diet high in whole grains, fiber, and fresh fruits and vegetables.
- Eat plenty of soy.
- Supplement your diet with one tablespoon of ground flaxseed or flaxseed oil a day.
- Avoid caffeine and minimize sugar and alcohol.
- Do not smoke.
- A good multivitamin/mineral with at least 50 milligrams of the B vitamins can help a lot.
- Take essential fatty acids in the form of evening primrose, black currant, or borage oils.
- Vitamin E, 400 to 800 IU, can often help decrease premenstrual breast swelling.
- Take calcium, 1,000 milligrams, and magnesium, 500 milligrams.
- Surround yourself with relaxing music and company (if you so desire), and take it easy.
- Avoid particularly stressful situations, confrontations, or decisions before your period.
- If your PMS is particularly intense, warn your partner in advance and give yourself space.
- Take some time out in nature or treat yourself to a favorite activity.
- For pelvic discomfort, take a sitz bath. Fill the tub with hot water up to two inches below your navel. Sit with your knees bent. Stay in the tub for five minutes. Then squat in a tub of cold water for one minute. Repeat the cycle two to three times.

	Key Symptoms	Mind	Body	Worse	Better	Food & Drink
Folliculinum *(Estrone/follicular hormone)*	Symptoms are worse from ovulation to menses Conditions begin after you take birth control pills Feel you have lost your sense of self Drained before your period	Feeling of being dominated Premenstrual depression Mood swings before period	Premenstrual headaches Premenstrual migraines Breasts swollen before period Ovulatory problems such as spotting and ovarian cysts	Heat Touch Noise	Fresh air	Extreme food cravings before your period
Kreosotum *(Creosote)*	Acrid, excoriating discharges Irritability Crumbling of the teeth Don't want to make love	Excited feeling premenstrually Fear of sexual assault Sensitivity to music You say you are well when you are very sick	Vaginal discharge before and after your period Burning vaginal discharge that irritates your labia Severe headache before and during your period Humming and buzzing sensations premenstrually	Making love Becoming chilled	Warmth Hot food	Desire for meat
Lachesis *(Bushmaster snake)*	You feel a huge sense of relief once you get your period Symptoms are worse on left side of body Symptoms move from left side to right You feel worse after sleep or on waking Intense symptoms and personality	Feel as if you will explode before your period Jealous and suspicious Very talkative Fear of snakes	Heavy, painful periods with clots You can't stand tight clothing around your neck or abdomen Can't even stand for the sheet to touch you at night You tend to sleep on your left side	After sleep Constriction of any kind Suppression of emotions or symptoms	Physical or emotional discharge	You desire coffee Desire oysters Worse from coffee during menopause
Lilium tigrinum *(Tiger lily)*	Very high sexual energy Uterine and ovarian problems You are compelled to keep busy Hurried	Strong religious interest combined with high sexual energy You feel wild and crazy Premenstrual irritability You must do several things at the same time	Intense vaginal itching before period Premenstrual breast tenderness Easily turned on Cutting pain in your abdomen premenstrually	Night Menses	Urinating Eating	You desire meat Aversion to food in general

Pulsatilla (Windflower)	Sepia (Cuttlefish ink)
Great medicine for hormonal problems	You feel crabby and put out before your period
All symptoms are changeable	No desire to make love
You are very emotional	Worn-out feeling
You hate getting overheated	Indifferent toward your partner and family

Crying before your period	You feel stuck
You love to be nurtured, comforted, and supported	Want to be left alone
Your nature is tender, warm, and affectionate	Cry easily
Need people around you	Love vigorous exercise and dancing

Exhausted before your period	Feel as if your uterus will fall out
Premenstrual yawning and stretching	Constipation worse before your period
Your digestion is worse before your period	Burning vaginal discharge
White or creamy vaginal discharge	Soreness, aching, and pressure in your abdomen

Being in a warm, stuffy room	Before your period
	Vinegar
	4:00 to 6:00 P.M.

Being outside	Vigorous exercise
Love and nurturing	Keeping busy

Desire for rich foods but feel worse after eating them	Desire for vinegar

155

Postpartum Depression (Mild)

Description

Postpartum depression, also called "blues," generally appears within the first day after delivery and lasts for weeks or sometimes longer. Your depression may be mild to severe.

Symptoms

You may experience sadness and a neutral feeling or a lack of desire to bond with your baby. You may feel regret or guilt about not being ecstatic after the birth. Other emotions may include hopelessness, a doubt about your ability to care for your child, mood swings, and a general feeling of being overwhelmed.

Complications

In rare cases, postpartum depression is so severe that the mother seeks to abandon or hurt the child.

Look

How am I responding to having just delivered my baby?
Is my behavior out of character?
Have I asked for anything in the way of help?
What is my interaction with my baby?

Listen

"I feel like I'm about to lose my mind." *Cimicifuga*
"I feel so exhausted that I don't know if I can handle my baby."
    Cypripedium
"I don't know why, but I want to cry." *Pulsatilla*
"I just want to be alone. Let someone else take care of the baby." *Sepia*

Ask

Do I feel anything unusual?
Do I have a sense that I can handle the situation?
How do I feel toward the baby?
Do I have any other symptoms?

Pointers for Finding Your Homeopathic Medicine

- If you find yourself sighing and your nerves are shot, consider *Cimicifuga*.
- *Cypripedium* is excellent for exhaustion and sleeplessness after childbirth.
- If you feel unusually needy and must have someone at your side, *Pulsatilla* is a good choice.
- *Sepia* is indicated if you experience an aversion toward your partner and, sometimes, your baby.

Dosage

- Take three pellets of 30C every three to four hours until you see an improvement.
- If you are no better after three doses, change medicines.
- After you first notice you have improved, take another dose only if your symptoms begin to return.
- Lower potencies (6X, 6C, and 30X) may need to be given more often (every one to two hours, depending on the severity of the symptoms).
- Higher potencies (200X, 200C, and 1M) usually need to be taken only once but may need a repetition if the symptoms are severe or return after initial improvement.

What to Expect

You should feel better within one week after taking the correct medicine. If you are not better within a couple of weeks, definitely seek out professional homeopathic care.

Women's Naturopathic Self-Care Recommendations

- Eat well for both of you, since you will, it is hoped, be nursing your baby very frequently. Eat lots of whole grains, organic fresh fruits and vegetables, fiber, and plenty of protein to keep up your energy.
- Drink at least six glasses of water a day.
- Avoid alcohol, caffeine, smoking, and excess sugar.
- Continue taking your prenatal vitamin/mineral as long as you are actively breastfeeding your baby. Make sure it contains 1,200 milligrams of calcium and 600 milligrams of magnesium, as well as at least 50 milligrams of B vitamins.
- Know that postpartum depression is common and you are not alone.

• Be sure to arrange for whatever help you need for the first couple of weeks after the birth.

• Take time to acknowledge your feelings honestly.

• Share your feelings honestly with your partner.

• Tap into your support system to get your needs met.

• Find a way to connect with other mothers of newborns.

• Get a massage or whatever makes you feel relaxed and special.

• If the feelings persist, don't hesitate to call a counselor so that the problem can be addressed promptly and you will be able to bond successfully with your baby.

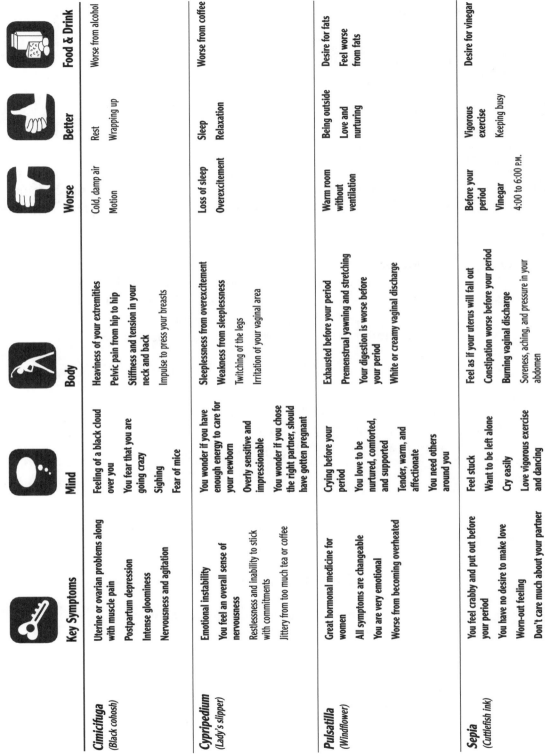

	Key Symptoms	Mind	Body	Worse	Better	Food & Drink
Cimicifuga (Black cohosh)	Uterine or ovarian problems along with muscle pain; Postpartum depression; Intense gloominess; Nervousness and agitation	Feeling of a black cloud over you; You fear that you are going crazy; Sighing; Fear of mice	Heaviness of your extremities; Pelvic pain from hip to hip; Stiffness and tension in your neck and back; Impulse to press your breasts	Cold, damp air; Motion	Rest; Wrapping up	Worse from alcohol
Cypripedium (Lady's slipper)	Emotional instability; You feel an overall sense of nervousness; Restlessness and inability to stick with commitments; Jittery from too much tea or coffee	You wonder if you have enough energy to care for your newborn; Overly sensitive and impressionable; You wonder if you chose the right partner, should have gotten pregnant	Sleeplessness from overexcitement; Weakness from sleeplessness; Twitching of the legs; Irritation of your vaginal area	Loss of sleep; Overexcitement	Sleep; Relaxation	Worse from coffee
Pulsatilla (Windflower)	Great hormonal medicine for women; All symptoms are changeable; You are very emotional; Worse from becoming overheated	Crying before your period; You love to be nurtured, comforted, and supported; Tender, warm, and affectionate; You need others around you	Exhausted before your period; Premenstrual yawning and stretching; Your digestion is worse before your period; White or creamy vaginal discharge	Warm room without ventilation	Being outside; Love and nurturing	Desire for fats; Feel worse from fats
Sepia (Cuttlefish ink)	You feel crabby and put out before your period; You have no desire to make love; Worn-out feeling; Don't care much about your partner and family	Feel stuck; Want to be left alone; Cry easily; Love vigorous exercise and dancing	Feel as if your uterus will fall out; Constipation worse before your period; Burning vaginal discharge; Soreness, aching, and pressure in your abdomen	Before your period; Vinegar; 4:00 to 6:00 P.M.	Vigorous exercise; Keeping busy	Desire for vinegar

Surgery *(Before and After)*

Description
Any type of operation, major or minor.

Symptoms
After surgery, you are bound to feel some pain, to a greater or lesser degree, depending on the type and extent of tissue or organs removed or repaired. Some types of surgery, particularly those involving the abdomen and pelvis, are often more painful and require a longer recovery.

Complications
One of the main complications following surgery is the development of scar tissue. Some scar tissue formation is a normal part of the postsurgical healing process, but the formation of adhesions can cause considerable pain, discomfort, and disfigurement, sometimes permanently.

Look
What does my scar look like? Size? Color?
Does it blanch when I press on it?
Are there any other visible symptoms?

Listen
"I just had a mastectomy, but no problem. I'll be just fine." *Arnica*
"I tried *Arnica* after surgery for prolapsed uterus, but it didn't help."
     Calendula
"I have shooting pains up my leg since undergoing heel surgery."
     Hypericum
"I still feel the after-effects of the anesthesia." *Phosphorus*
"My pelvic area is extremely sensitive since my hysterectomy."
     Staphysagria
"Ever since my fibroid was removed, I've been in a state of shock."
     Strontium carbonicum or *Arnica*

Ask

What is my particular type of surgery?

What are my symptoms?

Am I in pain? If so, what is the intensity, frequency, and type of pain?

What makes my pain better or worse?

How is my energy?

Have I felt any mental or emotional changes since the surgery?

What makes me feel better or worse overall?

Pointers for Finding Your Homeopathic Medicine

• The first medicine to take after surgery is *Arnica*.

• If *Arnica* doesn't help and there are no clear indications for the other medicines listed in this section, take *Calendula* internally.

• If you have shooting pain, numbness, or tingling following surgery, use *Hypericum*.

• *Phosphorus* can be very helpful if you feel woozy and disoriented even several days after surgery.

• After clean surgery of the abdominal organs where there is considerable sensitivity, consider *Staphysagria*.

• If you remain in a shocklike state after surgery, especially if you bled a lot, take *Strontium carbonicum*.

Dosage

• Take one dose of *Arnica,* 30C or 200C, the day before and the morning of your surgery and another dose as soon as you are awake following surgery. If you begin with *Arnica* 30C, continue taking it once a day until the pain is nearly or completely gone. If you are using a 200C potency, take another dose only if the pain returns. After two doses of *Arnica* 30C or one dose of *Arnica* 200C, if there are clear indications for one of the other medicines listed here, switch to that medicine.

• If you are no better after three doses of *Arnica* 30C or two doses of 200C, change medicines, if another fits your symptoms.

• After you first notice you have improved, take another dose only if your symptoms begin to return.

• Lower potencies (6X, 6C, and 30X) may need to be given more often (every two to four hours).

- Higher potencies (200X, 200C, and 1M) usually need to be taken only once but may need a repetition if the symptoms are severe or return after initial improvement.

What to Expect

Homeopathic medicines can help to speed up your healing process after surgery. I recommend this program for nearly any surgery, from dental surgery to a hysterectomy, with the exception of a very simple surgery, such as having a wart or mole removed. I recommend that you follow these suggestions for pre- and post-surgery, in addition to homeopathy, for the best results. I have used this program with hundreds of patients over the past sixteen years and, without exception, patients have healed rapidly and surgeons have remarked on how quickly and complication-free their recoveries were.

Women's Naturopathic Self-Care Recommendations

- As soon as you are allowed to eat or drink following surgery, begin taking a 250-mg capsule of bromelain three times a day. Continue taking these for three weeks. Note that bromelain capsules must be taken at least two hours away from eating any protein or they will merely act as an expensive digestive enzyme.
- Begin taking the following vitamins one week before surgery and continue for one month following surgery:

    Vitamin C (500 mg three times a day)

    Zinc (50 mg a day)

    Vitamin E (1,200 IU a day; if you have high blood pressure, take only 400 IU)

    Beta-carotene (50,000 IU per day)
- Apply *Calendula* and *Hypericum* tincture (diluted 1:3 parts) topically to prevent infection and to speed healing of the wound. (Do not apply *Arnica* topically if the skin is broken, such as after surgery, because it can cause a rash.)

	Key Symptoms	Mind	Body	Worse	Better	Food & Drink
Arnica (*Leopard's bane*)	Trauma, shock, surgery, and bleeding Bruising Post-surgery pain	Refuse help Say you are fine	**Bruising** Have cuts that bleed a lot **Want to lie down, but the bed feels too hard**	Touch Lying on a hard surface Motion	Lying down, especially with the head low	Craving for vinegar Aversion to milk and meat
Calendula (*Marigold*)	Clean surgical cuts Pain, bleeding	Fearful Nervous	Pain is out of proportion to the type of surgery	Chill	Lying still Walking around	Ravenous appetite
Hypericum (*St. John's wort*)	Surgery of nerve-rich areas, such as fingertips and toes Shooting pains, numbness, and tingling after surgery	Sad Mind feels dull Forget what you wanted to say	Infected wounds Gaping wounds Wounds resulting in weakness from loss of blood	Jarring the injured area Touch	Rubbing the area Lying on the face	Desire for pickles, wine and warm drinks
Phosphorus	Highly sensitive Tendency to bleed without clots Tremendous thirst for cold drinks You don't like being alone	**You are kindhearted and sympathetic** **Friendly and outgoing** **You pick up easily on others' feelings** You feel nervous before you go to a doctor	Woozy and disoriented days after anesthesia Persistent bleeding after surgery Burning pains Respiratory infections	Lying down Lying on the left side	Lying on your right side	**Great thirst for cold and carbonated drinks** **Desire for chocolate, salty, and spicy food**
Staphysagria (*Stavesacre*)	Wounds resulting from abdominal surgery of internal organs Area hypersensitive to the touch	Fear of doctors Sensitive to insults or rudeness Desire for advice or guidance	Stitching pains remaining after surgery	Touch Stretching the part	Rest	Desire for milk, bread, and tobacco
Strontium carbonicum (*Strontium carbonate*)	Shock after surgery Weakness after surgeries in which there was a lot of bleeding	Desire for advice or guidance	Fleeting pains Alternating pain and itching	Bleeding Uncovering	Wrapping up Hot bath or shower	Desire for bread and beer Aversion to meat

Vaginitis (Acute, not Recurrent)

Description

Vaginitis is an inflammation of the mucous membranes of your vagina. It may be caused by a viral, bacterial, trichomonal, or yeast infection or by sexual intercourse, douching, or other irritants such as spermicides, chemicals, or a foreign body in the vagina. If you are past menopause, you may experience atrophic vaginitis as a result of a decrease in your estrogen levels.

Symptoms

Vaginal discharge can be extremely annoying. It may be thick or thin, odorless or offensive. There may also be redness of the vaginal lips and itching, swelling, or pain of the vulva, labia, and vagina. The intensity varies greatly. In cases of severe vaginitis, you may find that sexual intercourse is so painful that it's not worth it.

Complications

A culture of your vaginal discharge can identify the cause of the infection. If gonorrhea, chlamydia, or syphilis are found to be the cause, the diagnosis must be reported to your local health department and immediate medical attention is required. AIDS testing may also be recommended, depending on your sexual exposure. If you have any of the three infections mentioned previously, you might have no symptoms at all, at least in the earlier stages. It is very important to be tested if you might have contracted these diseases, however, because if untreated, they can lead to infertility.

Look

Does my labia or vulva appear unusual?
Is there any swelling or discoloration?
Any eruptions?
If there is a vaginal discharge, what does it look like?

Listen

"I've never had such incredible itching in my whole life." *Caladium*
"My vagina burns so badly from the discharge that I can hardly stand it."
  Kreosotum
"I get this creamy discharge around my period. It makes me want to cry."
  Pulsatilla

"My vaginal discharge smells like old fish." *Sanicula*

"I got this yeast infection after my baby was born. I've had zero sex drive ever since." *Sepia*

Ask

When did my vaginal infection start?

Did something in particular seem to bring it on?

What are the main symptoms?

What makes them better or worse?

Is there any correlation between the vaginitis and sex?

Have I experienced any mental or emotional changes with the vaginitis?

Do I crave anything special to eat or drink?

Pointers for Finding Your Homeopathic Medicine

• For vaginitis with terrible itching during pregnancy, take *Caladium*.

• If your discharge is terribly acrid and excoriating, consider *Kreosotum*.

• For vaginitis with a yellowish-green, creamy discharge and if you are a sweet, sensitive woman who cries easily, you are likely to need *Pulsatilla*.

• *Sanicula* can be helpful if your discharge smells strongly like fish brine.

• If your symptoms occur during menopause and are accompanied by a loss of libido, constipation, and irritability, *Sepia* is probably your ticket.

Dosage

• Take three pellets of 30C every four hours until you see an improvement.

• If you are no better after three doses, change medicines.

• After you first notice you have improved, take another dose only if your symptoms begin to return.

• Lower potencies (6X, 6C, and 30X) may need to be given more often (every one to two hours, depending on the severity of the vaginitis).

• Higher potencies (200X, 200C, and 1M) usually need to be taken only once but may need a repetition if the symptoms are severe or return after initial improvement.

What to Expect

Acute episodes of vaginitis can respond within twenty-four to forty-eight hours but may take a week or two. Vaginitis is often a chronic or recurrent problem best treated by a professional homeopath.

Women's Naturopathic Self-Care Recommendations

• The easiest and most effective answer: Insert one capsule of boric acid powder vaginally in the morning and one capsule of acidophilus at bedtime for five days. Stop during your period.

• Douche with one tablespoon of white vinegar in a pint of warm water daily for five days. Insert one tablespoon of unsweetened, live-culture yogurt after each douche.

• If the vaginitis is only on the labia and vulva, rather than in the vagina, and is caused by yeast, apply a preparation of half vinegar and half water topically.

• Some women insert a clove of garlic, wrapped in cheesecloth or gauze, vaginally for yeast infections.

• If there is rawness externally *not* due to yeast, *Calendula* cream topically can be helpful.

• Insert vitamin E suppositories into the vagina for atrophic vaginitis.

• *Calendula* or vitamin A or herbal vaginal suppositories can be soothing. Occasionally, one tablespoon of baking soda in a quart of warm water works better as a douche than acidifying treatments such as vinegar or boric acid.

	Key Symptoms	Mind	Body	Worse	Better	Food & Drink
Caladium (American arum)	Terrible itching of the vagina Vaginitis during pregnancy	Nervous and excitable Restless after smoking Fearful of catching disease	Dryness of labia and vulva Itching of vagina and vulva with burning Desire to masturbate	Too much sex Tobacco	Cold air Sweating	Can only tolerate warm drinks
Kreosotum (Creosote)	Yellow vaginal discharge that is terribly itchy and burning Extreme rawness of the mucous membranes Discharge smells putrid or like green corn	Cross Obstinate Dissatisfied with everything	Swelling of the labia Scratching makes the itching and inflammation worse Vaginitis is worse during pregnancy or before the menstrual period starts Weakness of the legs	Pregnancy Menstrual period	Warmth Hot food Sitting	Crave smoked meat Aggravated by cold food
Pulsatilla (Windflower)	Thick, bland, yellow-green discharges Warm, with desire for fresh air or window open	Changeable emotions Clingy and weepy Want company when sick	Discharge may be bland, thick and milky, creamy or irritating, or thin and burning Discharge is usually painless Pain in the back and exhaustion with the discharge Lack of periods or late or irregular periods	Warm stuffy room Rich food	Slow walking in the open air	Not thirsty Desire for butter, ice cream, and creamy foods Aversion to and worse from fat, milk, and pork
Sanicula (Spring water)	Discharge smells like fish brine Body odor smells like old cheese	Stubborn, irritable, and touchy Don't want to be touched	Bearing-down sensation in the pelvis, as if uterus would drop out	Motion	Uncovering Rest	Desire for salt, bacon, and ice cold milk
Sepia (Cuttlefish ink)	Discharge makes your labia and vagina feel raw, burning, and itching Discharge is white or yellow and can be slimy, lumpy, or bloody Symptoms caused by a hormonal imbalance	Depressed, sluggish, dull, and overwhelmed Irritable Cry easily	Discharge worse during the day, none at night Dryness of the vagina in menopausal women that feels worse while walking Aversion to your partner and to sex Bearing-down sensation in the pelvis, as if uterus would fall out	Before the menstrual period Cold Pregnancy and after childbirth	Vigorous exercise or dancing Warmth Crossing legs	Desire for vinegar and sweets Aversion to fat

PART THREE

Homeopathic Care
from a Professional

What Every Woman Needs to Know About Homeopathic Treatment

What to Expect and What Will Be Expected of You

THE HOMEOPATHIC INTERVIEW

This section will give you a feeling for classical homeopathic treatment (sometimes called constitutional, meaning for your entire constitution). If you have never before consulted a homeopath, the first interview may surprise you. If you are used to having to blurt everything out quickly during a five- or ten-minute visit with your doctor before he leaves the room to move on to the next patient, this will be a very different experience. If you are accustomed to being asked a list of concrete questions about your physical symptoms and to answering with brief, concise replies, be ready for a change of pace.

A homeopath's office may or may not look like that of your regular doctor. Some homeopaths practice in medical office complexes with conventional practitioners. You may, however, find the office, as is the case in my practice, to be in a comfortable home setting. Depending on your practitioner's licensure and type of practice, there may or may not be other medical equipment present, such as an examination table. It is likely that your homeopath will sit in front of a computer or laptop or at least have those high-tech capabilities available at home where she studies her cases. Your homeopath will write down your case either by hand or on a computer but will try to record what you say as close to verbatim as possible.

Everything else I mention applies to both phone consultations and in-person office visits. You will have a minimum of an hour, probably an hour and a half or two, to say whatever you want about yourself. It is unlikely that your homeopath will interrupt you unless she wants to clarify something you have said, ask for an example, or inquire, "What else?" She will listen intently, perhaps with more interest and patience than any doctor you've ever seen before. If you need a few moments of silence to catch your train of thought, don't worry. It takes time to tell your life story and to make yourself understood thoroughly. Even if it takes several hours, the time is well spent. You see, everything you say is a reflection of your nature and can lead the homeopathic practitioner to find the right medicine for you. She will not settle for superficial answers and will probe, if necessary, to uncover your underlying feelings about your life and yourself. You may feel that she is asking you the same question in slightly different ways. She is only trying to understand the subtle ways in which you are unique and different from all of the other people in the world. It may seem to you that she is a bit slow on the uptake to be asking you so many questions that seem so obvious to you, but homeopaths are trained not to make any assumptions. What is true of one person may be just the opposite for the next.

WHAT A HOMEOPATH NEEDS TO KNOW ABOUT YOU

Anything that occurs to or interests you is likely to interest the homeopath who is taking your case. Feel free to start wherever you wish in talking about yourself. There should be enough time for you to share everything you want. Here are some important areas that can help her to understand you and select the best medicine:

- What brings you to seek out homeopathic care?
- When did each of your significant health problems begin and what was going on in your life at the time?
- What is your nature (temperament)?
- Who or what is most important to you?
- What have been the most difficult or upsetting times in your life?
- What situations do you find most unbearable?
- How did you feel during your childhood?
- What patterns or problems seem to have been with you throughout your life?
- What are your fears?
- What are your worries and concerns?
- Any recurrent thoughts or memories?
- What do you dream about at night (past and present)?
- What are the specific symptoms of your physical problems and what makes each better or worse?
- What would you change in your life if you could?
- Which of your parents are you most like?

- Which foods do you strongly like or dislike?
- How is your sleep?
- Do you tend to be warm or chilly?
- What other treatments are you receiving/have you received?
- If you have consulted a homeopath in the past, which medicines have and have not been effective?

The bottom line is that anything that makes you unique in any way can help your homeopath to help you. Let the interview flow naturally. Everything that is important will come out sooner or later.

THE HOMEOPATHIC PRESCRIPTION

After your initial appointment has ended, your homeopath will either prescribe a medicine for you to receive in the office or through a homeopathic pharmacy or will tell you she wishes to spend some time studying your case. In our practice, we prescribe at the time of the visit perhaps half the time and take the rest of our cases home for further study. Your homeopath may want to do a physical or laboratory examination or get the results of such an exam from your physician in order to obtain a pre-remedy assessment of your health status. You will be instructed about when and how to take the medicine. The dose you receive in the office or by mail may be the only medicine that is needed until your next appointment, or you may be given an additional homeopathic medicine to take on a regular basis.

The idea of one medicine encompassing all of your symptoms may be hard to grasp. You may ask, "Does this medicine treat my abnormal periods or my headaches? And what about my panic attacks?" Remember that the goal of homeopathy is to find one medicine for the whole person, so don't be surprised when your homeopath replies, "It's for all of you."

Some homeopaths have no qualms telling their patients which medicine they have chosen. Others would rather wait to give the full explanation until it is clear at the follow-up appointment that the chosen medicine is indeed the correct one. The only time it seems to matter a great deal is when someone is likely to read so much about the medicine that has been prescribed that the information presented at the next visit confuses or prejudices rather than informs the homeopath. Homeopaths try to remain unbiased and open-minded in thinking about what to give you and it is helpful if you do the same. On the other hand, I have had cases, particularly those of children, where the parent has made a suggestion of a homeopathic medicine based on what she read in one of our books, and it turns out that she is right on target.

If the first prescription is correct and you feel much better at your follow-up appointment six weeks or so later, it is likely, if you were given a single dose, that it will not be repeated unless your symptoms return. You will not need a different homeopathic medicine unless your symptoms shift substantially. If the first medicine you are given does not produce the desired changes, then your homeopath will change the prescription until he finds a medicine that produces significant and lasting improvement.

Although there are no actual side effects from homeopathic medicines, three types of reactions can occur:

• *An aggravation*—this is a temporary worsening of your already-existing symptoms, which rarely lasts for more than a few days (occasionally a couple of weeks) and generally indicates you have been given the correct homeopathic medicine.

• *A return of old symptoms*—this is a repetition of symptoms that you have had in the past, typically lasting for four to five days; it is thought to be a release of cellular patterning and only happens after you have taken the correct medicine.

• *A proving*—this is when, after taking a homeopathic medicine, you begin to notice new symptoms that you have not experienced in the past and that are known to be characteristic of the medicine you have taken. It is rare and generally happens only in extremely sensitive individuals or if you take the medicine too frequently.

THE TYPICAL COURSE OF TREATMENT

After your first appointment, you will be asked to schedule a follow-up appointment five to eight weeks later. At that time you will have a chance, usually for half an hour, to share everything that has changed or, it is hoped, improved, and everything that has not, as well as any new developments, dreams, circumstances, or perceptions. If you are doing well, you may not need another appointment for two to three months, depending on the protocol of your homeopath. If she has not yet found the right medicine, she will probably give you a different one and ask you to return again in five to eight weeks in order to evaluate your progress.

Once you are clearly on the right track as far as the choice of medicine, your appointments may be less frequent, every three to four or even six months apart, or on an as-needed basis. You will be asked to call or visit your homeopath if any acute illnesses arise that are severe or do not resolve on their own within a few days.

How long will you need to continue homeopathic care? This depends entirely on why you sought treatment in the first place, how well you have responded to homeopathic treatment, and whether you consider it to be a temporary experience on your path of healing or a type of treatment you wish to pursue long term. Many of my adult women patients consider homeopathy to be their medicine of choice for life. Whatever problems they may have, whether it be a car accident or a gall bladder attack or the grief of separation from a loved one, a pregnancy, or entering into menopause, they want to know how homeopathy can help. You will know, once you have experienced homeopathic treatment for a year or so, whether it is the type of natural medicine that will work for the rest of your life.

GIVE HOMEOPATHY A FAIR CHANCE

Suppose you have pursued homeopathic treatment with a practitioner for a year with little to no improvement? What next? A second opinion from another homeopath? Acupuncture? Conventional medicine? A chiropractor? Some cases are more challenging than others, and it may not be so easy to find a medicine that produces a profound effect. Here are some questions you can ask yourself in order to know what your next step should be:

* How do I feel about my relationship with my homeopath? Even though I haven't had a spectacular result from her treatment, do I feel that she is a healer for me? Does she understand me well? Do I feel at ease and able to communicate freely with her?
* How do I feel about homeopathy itself? Does it make sense? Does it seem like my path to healing?
* How experienced is my homeopath?
* Is there another treatment approach that really calls me now, or does it feel right to give homeopathy more time, either with my current homeopath or a different one?
* Are there additional changes I could make in my life to enhance my healing?

Once you've answered these questions, you will be clearer about what you want to do. If you have considerable trust in your homeopath, you may want to give it another six months or a year. So much new information has become available that, if your homeopath is actively searching out new medicines and approaches, she may be able to find a medicine she has not even previously considered. If you have confidence in homeopathy but not in your particular homeopath, request that she consult with or refer you to another, more experienced, homeopath. If it's time for you to try a new route, share this openly with your homeopath and she will probably give you her blessing to seek help elsewhere. What is most important is your healing, regardless of which path you take to get there.

ANTIDOTING SUBSTANCES TO AVOID DURING HOMEOPATHIC TREATMENT

Certain substances and procedures, according to many homeopaths, may interfere with the success of your treatment. How much they may affect you depends on many factors, but the primary factor is how sensitive you are to the substance and in general. Highly sensitive people often have to be more careful. I have seen many cases in which a woman did wonderfully for months after taking a particular homeopathic medicine and then, after exposure to one of the following, was back to square one or almost. I believe that the safest course is to avoid all of these influences, at least until it is obvious that a specific medicine has worked well for you. Then, if there is interference and the medicine needs to be repeated, at least your homeopath will be clear about what to give you. These are my guidelines; however, be sure to follow the recommendations of the homeopath you consult.

Avoid the Following, at Least Until It Is Clear Which Medicine You Need:

- Coffee in any form (including decaf and coffee-flavored desserts)
- Products containing strong aromatic substances such as camphor, eucalyptus, menthol, tea tree, pine oil, and phenol (this includes BENGAY, Carmex, Blistex, Vicks, Ricola, Chapstick, Tiger Balm, many liniments and mouthwashes, cleaning products such as Lysol and Pine-Sol, and others, so you need to read labels carefully). These substances most consistently antidote homeopathic medicine.
- Electric blankets
- Hair permanents
- Dental drilling, anesthetic, and ultrasonic cleaning (your practitioner can advise you about the best time to schedule dental work so that it is least likely to interfere with your treatment)

WHEN TO CALL OR SEE YOUR HOMEOPATH

It is important to keep your homeopath abreast of what is happening with you and your health. Let her know if there are any significant changes, any disturbing symptoms, serious acute illnesses that don't resolve on their own, or significant life traumas. Be sure to advise her if the medicine does not seem to help you or if you began to feel quite well, then relapsed. Sometimes women leave homeopathic treatment out of frustration, when the solution is as simple as taking a higher dose of the medicine that she has already been prescribed. If I don't hear from a patient who is doing well, I assume that she is continuing to feel quite good unless she lets me know otherwise. If that's not the case and she is dissatisfied with her progress, I can do nothing to help her unless I know exactly what's going on. At times, my patients are reluctant to call me over the weekend, even though they know I carry a pager. I, and most other homeopaths, would much rather help my patients with an acute illness early on instead of waiting until the illness has progressed, they have gone through unnecessary suffering, and they might have resorted to conventional medicine. Homeopathy can be very powerful in rapidly and effectively treating acute illnesses in a way that strengthens, rather than suppresses, your immune system.

WHAT WOMEN ASK ME ABOUT HOMEOPATHIC TREATMENT

Some questions are bound to come up as you think more about what you have read in this book. Here are the most frequently asked questions about homeopathic treatment, and I refer you to *The Patient's Guide to Homeopathic Medicine: What You Need to Know to Make the Most of Your Treatment and Care,* if you have more concerns. If you are strictly interested in treating yourself for acute conditions, the self-care section of this book should answer most questions that arise.

- *What are the chances that homeopathy can help me?* Of course, your prognosis with homeopathy depends on a number of factors, including your diagnosis, overall state of health, mental attitude, lifestyle, and so forth. For many of the conditions in this book, I estimate a 70 percent success rate if you continue with treatment for at least a year, although the positive results for most women will begin within a month or two after taking the correct medicine.

- *How can homeopathy help if my problems are hormonal?* Hormonal imbalances are a result of the overall imbalance in you as a whole. Once that imbalance is corrected, the endocrine system as well as all of the other organs and systems of your body will fall into place, along with your energy, mental abilities, creativity, and emotional well-being.

- *Can I still be treated homeopathically if I choose to take hormones or fertility drugs?* Yes. Since a homeopath will evaluate all of your symptoms rather than just your hormonal functioning, she should still be able to tell when she has found the medicine for you. Once that happens and you feel better, you may choose to make a different decision regarding your drugs. However, even if you continue taking hormone replacement indefinitely, homeopathy can still work.

- *What if I have other physical problems like headaches or asthma?* One medicine really can treat all of you. The same medicine that improves your gynecological symptoms should also help your headaches and asthma substantially.

- *Can I really find an alternative to antibiotics for my bladder infections?* Not only should homeopathy be able to help you through your acute bladder infections without your having to resort to antibiotics, but it should prevent future bladder infections, or at least diminish their frequency and severity. I also make other recommendations for bladder infections in addition to homeopathy, as you will see on pages 192 and 193.

- *Can homeopathy also help for depression and anxiety?* Homeopathy is unquestionably the best therapy I have ever found for depression, anxiety, and other mental and emotional problems. The effects are lasting, you will not suffer the side effects of conventional psychiatric medications, and healing occurs at the deepest possible level. Please see *Prozac-Free: Homeopathic Medicine for Depression, Anxiety, and Other*

Mental and Emotional Problems for much more information and numerous case studies from our practice.

- *Are homeopathic medicines really safe during pregnancy?* Homeopathy is completely safe during pregnancy, more so than herbs. If, however, a miscarriage is imminent, homeopathy will most likely not prevent it from occurring.

- *What about using homeopathy while I nurse my baby?* Homeopathic medicines are perfectly safe during pregnancy, while nursing, and for newborns. I have treated one-day-old babies with homeopathy.

- *Can I use homeopathy during my delivery?* Yes. Homeopathy has been known to work miracles during deliveries. You need to clear it with your midwife or physician prior to the delivery and should consider including such wishes in your birth plan.

- *Do I have to stop taking my vitamins?* There is no problem with taking most vitamins and minerals while being treated homeopathically. However, it is not necessary or desirable while doing homeopathy to take so many supplements that your symptoms are masked. Some homeopaths advise against taking nutritional supplements, but, perhaps because I am a naturopathic physician trained in nutrition, I am not one of them. I consider these supplements to be part of your insurance policy for health and longevity.

- *Will homeopathy help me lose weight?* Homeopathy, by itself, will only occasionally promote weight loss, such as when your underfunctioning thyroid is reactivated and your metabolism is given a jump-start. But I see frequently that once a woman feels more energetic, positive, and healthy, she is far more motivated to do whatever is necessary to modify her diet and lifestyle to lose weight.

- *Can I use homeopathy as my only treatment to prevent osteoporosis?* I would not feel comfortable with using homeopathy exclusively during postmenopause. There is too much evidence concerning the importance of diet, exercise, and nutritional supplements such as calcium and, as far as I know, no scientific research on the use of homeopathy alone in the prevention of osteoporosis.

- *If I am already being treated for breast cancer, how can homeopathy help?* Homeopathy can still help you in a number of ways: to strengthen your vital force and immune system, heal all of your other symptoms, improve your overall state of well-being, and decrease your likelihood of a recurrence. As with osteoporosis prevention, I also recommend an integrated program of diet, supplements, exercise, lifestyle, and attitudinal healing for cancer.

- *I've already had two surgeries for endometriosis and have taken every drug in the book. Can homeopathy help?* I have found homeopathy to be extremely effective for endometriosis, far more than anything else I have seen. I would highly recommend it before trying more surgeries or hormones.

- *None of my doctors can figure out why I continue to miscarry. Is there any chance of keeping a pregnancy with homeopathy?* It is not necessary to know the cause of the miscarriages for homeopathy to work. If your organs are intact and there is nothing that absolutely prevents you from becoming pregnant, I would urge you to give homeopathy at least a year to help you keep a pregnancy to full term and deliver a healthy baby.

- *My fibroid is growing and causing excessive urination and bleeding. What can homeopathy offer?* I would estimate that over 90 percent of the women I have treated for uterine fibroids have not gone on to have hysterectomies. The bleeding, frequent urination, and pain are generally handled with homeopathy. It is rare that the fibroid actually shrinks, but its size is usually kept at bay until menopause, when, due to decreased estrogen production, the growth tends to no longer be a problem.

- *I've tried to get pregnant for four years. I would not want more than one baby, and I just don't feel comfortable with fertility drugs. What are the odds of homeopathy helping me get pregnant?* There are no statistics on how often homeopathy works for infertility. My experience is mostly with endometriosis, and the outcomes are often positive. It is definitely worth giving homeopathy a year or two, if you are willing to take the time, before undergoing more invasive procedures.

- *How will I know if the homeopathic treatment is working?* It will be very obvious to you and your practitioner. I expect a minimum of a 70 percent improvement in most symptoms, and usually 80 percent or more, after at least six weeks. This, of course, depends on your diagnosis and situation, but your results will *not* be too subtle to tell whether the medicine is working.

- *How long will it take to start feeling better?* You may feel better within days, and a few of my patients feel better almost instantly, but you need to allow at least five or six weeks to evaluate yourself after taking a homeopathic medicine. If your chief complaint has to do with your periods, I suggest that you go through two full periods before evaluating the effect of the medicine.

- *Do homeopathic medicines have side effects like regular drugs?* No. You do not need a *Physicians Desk Reference (PDR)* for homeopathy. However, aggravations (a transient worsening of already-existing symptoms), and a return of old symptoms (a brief recurrence of symptoms long past) can occur as part of the healing process. A third phenomenon, called a proving, is rare, and involves your experiencing new symptoms that are characteristic of the medicine. All three of these pass relatively quickly (with a proving, you need to stop taking the medicine). There is no such thing as an allergic reaction to a homeopathic medicine.

- *Are homeopathic medicines prescription or over-the-counter?* Homeopathic medicines sold in the United States are regulated by the FDA. Most are over-the-counter and a few are restricted to physicians.

- *Can I begin homeopathy while I am still under conventional treatment?* Absolutely. We see many patients who are taking pharmaceuticals when they begin homeopathic treatment. In many cases, depending on the circumstances, patients can discontinue their medications under their doctors' guidance as they get well. This is generally not true, though, of medications such as long-term thyroid supplementation, insulin for diabetes, and long-standing antipsychotic medications for schizophrenia.

- *How often will I have to see or talk to my homeopath?* At the beginning I see patients every six to eight weeks. Once you are doing well, your visits will likely be every three, four, or even six months.

- *How long will I have to be under homeopathic care?* Plan on a minimum of a year or two. Many women are so pleased with homeopathic care that they continue using it for life.

- *How expensive is it to see a homeopath?* Fees vary, depending on experience and location. First visits generally range from $200 to $500, with beginning homeopaths more on the low end, and return visits from $75 to $150. The medicines themselves cost next to nothing. A year's supply of homeopathic medicine generally costs far less than a month's worth of a single pharmaceutical drug.

- *Is homeopathy covered by health insurance?* In some cases, yes; however, many homeopaths, for a variety of reasons, including protection of patient confidentiality, prefer to stay out of the managed care system.

- *How long a time should I give homeopathy to help me?* At least one year, but it may, in some cases, take two to three years to be helped if your case is complicated. It is important to continue with treatment at least until you are significantly better and stable, on all levels. Some of the deepest and lasting changes, such as the dissolution of a limiting, underlying pattern, may take even five years or more, but it is well worth being patient to produce such a dramatic shift.

- *How can I find a qualified homeopath in my area?* There are several directories of homeopathic practitioners. See the appendix of this book. Some homeopaths, such as myself, will do long-distance telephone consultations, particularly when there are no experienced practitioners in your area.

CHAPTER 13

Conditions for Which You Need a Homeopath

HOW TO BEST USE THIS CHAPTER

The conditions listed in this chapter fall into the category of chronic women's problems, physical, mental, and emotional, that are simply too complex to lend themselves to self-treatment. In addition to gynecological conditions, I have included other problems that are quite common to women, such as depression, anxiety, hormonally related headaches, and eating disorders. The section is limited to the most common women's problems that I have seen. If you have a more unusual women's condition, please consult a homeopath. Even if there is no experienced homeopathic practitioner in your vicinity, some of us are quite agreeable to treating patients by phone, in which case you would receive any necessary physician's examinations locally. Almost *any* condition that you might have can potentially benefit from homeopathic treatment, regardless of whether it is included here. I have also indicated, based on my clinical experience, just how likely homeopathy is to help you for your specific problem, as well as other naturopathic therapies that can go hand in hand quite nicely with homeopathy.

This section of the book is meant to familiarize you with the possibilities of homeopathic treatment, as well as with some of my cases and the candid personal experiences (all names have been changed) of some of my patients. Through their words, you can get a first-hand feeling for what women with various problems will likely go through and gain from homeopathy.

I do *not* include much of the valuable information contained in more broadly focused books on alternative health care for women, such as anatomy, physiology, and specific diets and recipes. An excellent source of this type of information are Dr. Susan Lark's many books on specific women's conditions (see appendix). I heartily encourage you to become as familiar as possible with women's health in general and your own body-mind in particular, but the emphasis of my book is on how homeopathy can help you. I also do not cover what type of testing is recommended to accurately diagnose each condition, but that information is readily available in other women's books and through your physician. I list many other wonderful books on women's health care in the appendix.

These icons appear in this chapter:

Description
Defines the condition and what causes it.

Symptoms
Describes the common symptoms of the condition.

Complications
Tells you about potential problems, medical emergencies, and when you need medical assistance.

Conventional Treatment
Describes how the condition is treated by conventional medicine.

What to Expect from Homeopathic Treatment
Gives you a realistic time frame for getting better.

Naturopathic Suggestions to Complement Homeopathic Care
Offers other natural and practical tips to help and support you.

Acne Rosacea

Julie's Story

"I started homeopathic treatment with Dr. Reichenberg-Ullman nearly a year after she began treating my ten-year-old son for oppositional-defiant disorder. She's advised us both by phone because we live in another state. His behavior improved considerably, but that didn't take away my extreme frustration and irritability. I found myself in an almost constant state of anxiety over everything that I couldn't seem to complete to my level of satisfaction. Foggy-headedness and forgetfulness had definitely interfered with my ability to accomplish what I wanted.

"My most troubling physical problem was a skin condition called rosacea that came upon me shortly after my son's birth and got steadily worse. A dermatologist prescribed oral antibiotics and a topical ointment, which did help, but he told me I'd need to continue for life and the idea of being on a steroidal preparation forever did not appeal to me. It seemed like it was just a way to suppress the problem rather than address the root cause. The antibiotics caused me to develop a vaginal yeast infection, for which he simply prescribed more drugs. When I inquired about taking acidophilus, he told me it was unproven and would do no good. I felt worse by the day. This is when I decided to be treated homeopathically myself, which is one of the best decisions I have ever made.

"Other problems that I hoped would improve with homeopathy were my nervousness around people; my PMS, which has gotten progressively worse over the past ten years since my daughter was born; heavy periods; and zero sex drive. And, if some miracle were possible, I also longed for help with poor concentration, unreasonable anger, and a tendency to become chilled, especially my legs and feet.

"Looking back, I can honestly say that my relationships with my husband and kids were a chaotic wreck. But, underneath it all, we had a lot of love and I never gave up hope and prayers.

"I stopped using my topical medication for the rosacea before I took the homeopathic medicine. My dermatologist had warned me that my skin would become immediately worse but, to my pleasant surprise, it didn't. In fact, once I started homeopathy, the rosacea went away and never came back except for once, briefly, after I was exposed to aromatherapy. My vaginal infection disappeared as well.

"At one point during my homeopathic treatment, I became much angrier, felt incredibly jealous toward my husband for no reason at all, and cried as if my heart would break. It felt like a release of old, suppressed pain and memories from a past abusive relationship. It was as if I had this intense desire to bring everything out into the open . . . all the things I'd kept inside for so many years. I compared it to a dam breaking. Most amazing to me is that during this outpouring of emotions, my head began to feel clearer and more focused, I stopped forgetting everything, and my heart stopped aching.

"Then, remarkably, my sexual energy came back for the first time in ten years. I even let my house get messy while I put more energy into healing our marriage. This was very unlike the me who could not seem to relax unless everything was just so. I also have lots more energy and enjoy exercising again. My annoying toenail fungus is even slowly going away after almost four years of it being so bad that my nail almost fell off.

"This has been a wonderful experience for me and for my family. Homeopathy is amazing medicine."

I gave Julie *Crotalus cascavella* (Brazilian rattlesnake) because of her impatience, tendency to rush all the time, rosacea, difficulty trusting others because she felt they talked behind her back, fear of rattlesnakes and copperheads, recurrent dreams of snakes, and the feeling of having to hide from her alcoholic father as a child.

Julie has needed two doses of the *Crotalus* during her nine months of treatment and she cannot say enough wonderful things about the change in her. Her acne rosacea is dramatically better, her vaginitis is gone, her sexual energy has returned after a two-year absence, she feels calmer, her memory has improved significantly, she is less frustrated and anxious, and her overall attitude is much more positive.

Description
Rosacea is a chronic, inflammatory skin disease that usually begins in middle age or later and is more likely to be a problem if you have a fair complexion.

Symptoms
You will notice redness and flushing of the nose and cheeks, broken blood vessels, and small, pus-filled eruptions.

Complications
Secondary infections, but mostly, embarrassment.

Conventional Treatment
Topical metronidazole (Flagyl) gel or broad-spectrum oral antibiotics (generally tetracycline) are most commonly prescribed. Retin-A is used in more difficult cases.

What to Expect from Homeopathic Treatment

Rosacea can definitely be helped with homeopathy, as you learned from the dramatic response in Julie's case, but it can sometimes be a challenge.

Naturopathic Suggestions to Complement Homeopathic Care

- Avoid hot, spicy food and hot drinks.
- Acid fruit can often aggravate rosacea.
- Avoid coffee, tea, alcohol, and smoking.
- Take a high-quality megamultivitamin and mineral.
- Some women find large doses of B-vitamins, particularly riboflavin, to be helpful.
- Drink at least six glasses of water a day.
- Birth control pills may cause or aggravate the problem.

Acne Vulgaris

Jamie's Story

"I started seeing Judyth eight years ago when I was in high school for a number of reasons: I was sick way too often, had acne, and was often depressed. I had spent a good portion of my life on antibiotics and fighting off colds and bronchitis every year. Fortunately, my parents were open to alternative forms of medicine.

"My first office visit was different from any doctor's appointment I'd ever had before. I remember telling friends afterward that it was more like what I imagined going to a psychologist would be. Along with asking me about any physical symptoms, Judyth was interested in my sleeping habits, what kinds of foods I craved or disliked, what my worst fears were, and so on. I was amazed when she started telling me things about myself that she had figured out, based on the homeopathic medicine she felt I needed.

"The first six months are sketchy in my memory. My acne became worse as it worked its way out of my system. I have to admit, it was really hard for me to have my entire face covered with acne, but I stuck it out. I kept thinking, "Just get it all out of your system now and you won't have to deal with it anymore. No more pills, no more zit creams, no more dermatologists. If this works, it will be worth it."

"I initially felt worse but, as every patient learns, this is often the first step to getting better. Pretty soon, I went through my first winter ever of not being sick! My acne still was present to a small degree, but I felt really good. The acne was never again a significant problem. And I have stayed healthy since."

For the past six and a half years *Natrum muriaticum* has helped Jamie consistently, not only with her acne. Sensitive, artistic, and idealistic, Jamie marches to her own drumbeat. Because she is a great listener, her friends know they can come to her regularly for a shoulder to cry on, and they do so frequently. Watching Jamie blossom from a young woman of sixteen who was just beginning to define her own identity to a talented, creative, and self-reliant woman of twenty-three has been a delight.

Description

You may have thought that once you survived the tempestuous teenage years, your skin would be creamy and clear. But facial acne, an inflammation of the hair follicles and sebaceous glands and colloquially called pimples or zits, is often associated with fluctuating hormones. It may, consequently, become exacerbated premenstrually, during pregnancy (at which time it may also disappear), or during menopause, as well as if you take birth control pills.

Symptoms

Acne can run the gamut of superficial, mild blemishes to deep, cystic, inflamed, scarring lesions. These may take the form of open (blackheads) or closed (whiteheads) eruptions, as well as inflamed papules, pustules, or cysts.

Complications

Other than the risk of secondary bacterial infections, the most distressing complication of acne is the effect it can have on your self-esteem.

Conventional Treatment

The most common conventional treatments, depending on the extent and severity of the lesions, include benzoyl peroxide, topical antibiotic solutions, retinoic acid (Retin-A), natural or artificial sunlight, and oral antibiotics. Be aware of the side effects, especially during pregnancy.

What to Expect from Homeopathic Treatment

Homeopathy is often effective for acne, especially in combination with nutritional supplementation, herbs, and, in some cases, dietary changes. Your homeopath may recommend discontinuing conventional drugs, such as oral and topical antibiotics, before beginning homeopathic treatment of acne, since these drugs can be suppressive. I have not found benzoyl peroxide to interfere with homeopathic care.

Naturopathic Suggestions to Complement Homeopathic Care
- Eat a low-fat, whole-foods diet that is high in whole grains, fresh fruits and vegetables, fiber, soy, and flax.
- Drink at least six glasses of water a day.
- Avoid coffee, tea, alcohol, and tobacco.
- Eliminate or minimize those foods that clearly aggravate your skin.
- Use *Calendula* soap.
- Use green clay or bentonite clay packs twice a week.
- Take black currant, evening primrose oil, or borage oil.
- Take a high-quality megamultivitamin and mineral, including vitamin A or beta-carotene, 50,000 IU; vitamin E, 400 to 1,000 IU; zinc, 30 to 50 milligrams; and vitamin C, 1,000 to 2,000 milligrams.
- Indulge in hot water steams (avoid aromatherapy with homeopathy!).
- Herbs, including Oregon grape, dandelion root, burdock, and *Calendula,* can be taken in a tincture form.
- Cultivate a regular routine of aerobic exercise.

Anxiety

Christine's Story

"I have used homeopathy for years. When I lived in New York, despite the fact that naturopathic doctors could not be licensed there, I sought relief from heavy bleeding and clotting during perimenopause and countless other day-to-day ailments that cropped up in our family. Thanks to a regimen of homeopathy and vitamins, I made it through that time without surgery or drugs. But my most dramatic homeopathic success story occurred years later after we had moved to Seattle.

"My son, at age fifteen, showed signs of an emerging mental illness. At first I attributed it to his being a teenager, but it became apparent that it was more. We took our son in for homeopathic treatment and, over the next year and a half, he was more stable. Eventually, due to the seriousness of his problem, we ended up with a combination of drugs and homeopathy that has worked quite well. Homeopathy enables us to keep the drug dosage to a minimum.

"This was an incredibly stressful time. There is no history of mental illness in our family and I just couldn't believe my wonderful son had been so afflicted. One night the burden of his care came crashing down on my shoulders. I felt faint and could not breathe. When I went to bed, I asked my husband to please check on me periodically and, if I still was unable to breathe, that he take me to the local emergency room.

"It then became clear that I, as well as my son, needed treatment just to get through such a challenging time. I found the initial homeopathic interview to be much like a therapy session, with me blurting out my feelings through a myriad of Kleenex tissues. When I calmed down, I began to answer more general questions.

"As a side note, I mentioned my tendency to become seasick very easily. That was apparently of great homeopathic interest. As long as I can remember, being in any stuffy place, let alone on a boat, plane, or carnival ride, rocked my equilibrium to the point of my almost fainting. Sometimes even bending over would cause me to feel some imaginary wave, as if my feet were not on solid ground.

"Although it was anxiety and a type of nervous exhaustion that led me to Dr. Reichenberg-Ullman, she put all of my symptoms together. That led her to prescribe *Cocculus*. Under the description of a patient needing this medicine, she described, 'One who is caring for and losing sleep over a sick loved one.' Bingo. That, plus the motion sickness and a feeling of being wrung-out, fit me perfectly.

"The *Cocculus* helped calm me and kept my head level while I managed my son's illness. I slept better and felt more hopeful and peaceful. The changes were subtle and it wasn't until several weeks later that I realized that the woozy, rocking sensation that had plagued me had vanished altogether. One dose of the medicine lasted almost a year. I am grateful to report that my son is doing very well, and so am I."

Christine has described her own case and the indications for *Cocculus* (Indian cockle) quite well. It is an excellent medicine for motion sickness, along with anxiety and nervous exhaustion after caring for or losing sleep over worrying about a loved one.

Women like Christine who need this medicine are quite sensitive to the needs of others, often at the expense of their own. *Cocculus* is also quite a common homeopathic answer to morning sickness. Since I began to see Christine four years ago, she has needed six doses of *Cocculus* in a 200C potency, as well as infrequent, self-administered doses of a 30C.

Barbara's Story

"When I called Dr. Reichenberg-Ullman, I had experienced a myriad of symptoms for many years. I didn't always feel bad; they seemed to come and go. But, since the birth of my second child seven years ago, I seemed to worsen. The symptom that bothered me the most was anxiety. I was afraid of the dark and of bug bites. I would have these little spells where I would get a rush of adrenaline and my throat would feel tight, as if I would not be able to swallow. This would last anywhere from five minutes to half an hour. It could occur at any time and in any place. There seemed to be no reason.

"Once I was hospitalized for anxiety and depression. They told me I needed a good rest. I was put on antidepressants for these conditions and was told I would need them for the rest of my life. I had a hard time accepting these diagnoses because, when I feel well, I am a very positive person and far from depressed.

"Homeopathy makes so much sense to me because it gets to the root of the problem, rather than calling it a disease and merely treating the symptoms. Since starting homeopathic treatment, I no longer take anything for anxiety or depression. I feel much quieter inside. I feel as if I could write for days about how much I believe that homeopathy works. It's not a quick fix but it is well worth the time and patience that it has taken for me to feel well again."

The medicine that helped Barbara with her anxiety was *Apis mellifica* (honeybee), prescribed on the basis of her anxiety about her family and hives and anaphylaxis (severe, life-threatening allergic reaction) following a bumblebee sting as a child. Twice more, she was unable to breathe and went into shock after bug bites. *Apis* also fit Barbara's industrious nature and desire to protect her family from any danger, as well as her premenstrual irritability (cross as a bee). The medicine that followed *Apis,* in Barbara's case, was *Phosphorus.*

Description
Anxiety is a feeling of nervousness, restlessness, and general apprehension, sometimes characterized by acute episodes of panic.

Symptoms
You may have a sense of uneasiness, fear, dread, or terror, along with one or more of the following: rapid heart rate, heart pain or palpitations, hyperventilation, trembling, butterflies in the stomach, constipation, nausea, diarrhea, fatigue, headaches, sleeplessness, tendency to startle, dizziness, and a sense of unreality.

Complications
Severe anxiety can result in hospitalization and significant, sometimes permanent, limitations on your life.

Conventional Treatment

Anti-anxiety medications, antidepressants, psychotherapy, and relaxation techniques.

What to Expect from Homeopathic Treatment

Homeopathy can produce excellent long-term results and can often eliminate the need for conventional medications.

Naturopathic Suggestions to Complement Homeopathic Care

• Limit your focus to the present moment. Avoid obsessing about what happened in the past and what may or may not ever happen in the future.
• Alternate nostril breathing just before bedtime can be extremely beneficial. Close off your right nostril with your right thumb pressed against the side of your nose. Inhale slowly through your left nostril. With your middle finger, close off your left nostril, release your thumb to open your right nostril, and exhale. Inhale through the right nostril. Now close off the right nostril and exhale through the left. Inhale slowly through the left and switch again, exhaling through the right. Continue for three to ten minutes.
• Take a peaceful walk in nature.
• Gently remind yourself that worrying doesn't change anything for the better and can make you miserable in the meantime.
• Take Bach Flower Rescue Remedy, five drops under the tongue, up to several times a day.
• Regular exercise gets those endorphins flowing.
• Get involved in volunteer or service activities that take your mind off of your problems.

Bladder Infections and Problems (Recurrent)

Shanti's Story

"My first attack of cystitis happened following a bladder infection while I enjoyed a vacation in Hawaii. After returning home, the symptoms persisted until I ended up at the urologist's office, where he dilated my urethra. The problem seemed to clear up—

until the next time! All of my subsequent attacks had one thing in common: no infection was ever again cultured. I believe that my intense pain, spasm, cramping, and frequent and painful urination fit the description of interstitial cystitis (IC). Unfortunately, the only way to confirm the diagnosis is by bladder biopsy, something I was not eager or willing to do.

"I found a second urologist who gave me a new approach to handling my problem, mainly through some dietary changes, and it did help. But I continued to have recurrent episodes and each time they lasted longer and longer.

"My family practice doctor suggested homeopathy as a more permanent approach. Soon after Dr. Reichenberg-Ullman gave me a constitutional homeopathic medicine, the pain diminished rapidly. I could finally sleep without depending on pain medications and no longer feared gong to the bathroom because it didn't hurt anymore. Thanks to homeopathy, I became pain-free. Homeopathic medicine literally changed the quality of my life. I truly believe that other women in my position can be helped, too."

Chronic bladder infections often respond beautifully to homeopathic treatment. Shanti's case of interstitial cystitis is a chronic, noninfectious bladder problem for which conventional medicine has no sure cure. Shanti only needed homeopathic treatment for a year and a half. During her severe episodes of interstitial cystitis, the cramping in her bladder was nearly unbearable, regardless of her position. Also of concern were burning in the urethra, a constant awareness of her bladder, severe uterine cramping during her periods, mood swings, and breasts so painful that lying face down was an ordeal. After taking *Cascarilla* (gallow grass), the urgency and cramping were gone and her periods were much improved as were her other symptoms.

Description

Bladder infections, also known as cystitis or urinary tract infections (UTIs), are fifty times more prevalent in women between the ages of twenty and fifty. Many women get them at some point in their lives.

Symptoms

The most common symptoms are pain in the urethra (where the urine comes out) or bladder before, during, or after urination, and urinary urgency and frequency. You may have blood in your urine and may suffer some lower back pain (which can be a red flag for a kidney infection). Bladder infections vary in intensity and onset, from excruciating and sudden pain to milder and more tolerable discomfort of more gradual onset. You may have no apparent symptoms even though your bacterial culture is positive, or you may experience symptoms without any evidence of infection. You are more likely to get a bladder infection after sex with a new partner, after having postponed urination, after having become dehydrated, or following catheterization. Sexually transmitted diseases can also be a cause of chronic urinary infections. Interstitial cystitis, though not an infection per se, features many of the symptoms of a bladder infection, but bacterial cultures tend to be normal.

Complications

Your biggest risk is of the bladder infection ascending up your ureter (the tube going from the bladder to the kidney), resulting in acute pyelonephritis, a serious infection of the kidneys. Urinary frequency, urgency, and pain, accompanied by pain along the sides of the mid-back and fever, can indicate pyelonephritis, in which case you need immediate medical attention.

Conventional Treatment

Antibiotics are the allopathic treatment of choice.

What to Expect from Homeopathic Treatment

Homeopathy has an excellent track record in helping to eliminate urinary infections or making them much less severe and frequent.

Naturopathic Suggestions to Complement Homeopathic Care

- Drink at least six glasses of water a day on an ongoing basis.
- If you have a tendency to recurrent bladder infections, you may want to take cranberry concentrate or capsules on a regular basis to acidify your urine. Cranberry juice is adequate if that is all you have available, but the sugar content is high. Once you have been on an effective homeopathic medicine for a couple of months, you can generally discontinue the cranberry supplements.
- Go to the bathroom as soon as you feel the urge. Do *not* put it off.
- Urinate after you make love.
- During an infection, take bladder herbs such as Oregon grape, *Bucchu, Pipsissewa, Uva ursi,* and cornsilk every two hours until your symptoms improve. The dosage will depend on whether you take them in the form of a tea, capsules, or tincture.

- If you tend to develop a bladder infection from getting chilled, bundle up and stay warm.
- Some women find that citrus fruits aggravate their cystitis. If so, avoid them.

Breast Cancer

My Own Story

The diagnosis of ductal carcinoma in situ (DCIS) took me quite by surprise. I was the only one in my circle of friends to get breast cancer. What became exceedingly clear to me right off was that I wanted, if possible, to live a long, healthy life. My parents lived to eighty-seven and eighty-nine, and I wasn't ready to die at fifty. I had seen some women who put all of their faith in natural medicine die of breast cancer, and, being a naturopathic doctor, I wanted the best of both worlds. When I was told that my particular type of breast cancer was noninvasive and that with a mastectomy there would be a 98 percent chance that the cancer would not return later in the same breast, the odds sounded pretty good. No chemotherapy or radiation was even recommended for DCIS.

I did a lot of things very quickly. I found two surgeons in whom I had great confidence. I contacted a woman homeopath in India and asked her to take me on as a patient, found a wonderful spiritual healer (actually two), and got a great deal of support from my friends and, most of all, my husband. I was already taking a ton of supplements and had changed my diet dramatically a year before to the Zone. Turns out, the cancer had been developing for six or seven years.

Not everyone agreed with all of my decisions, even my husband. But I knew inside that I was immensely fortunate to have a noninvasive rather than an invasive type of breast cancer, which would require my facing the difficult choice of whether or not to have radiation and/or chemotherapy.

The surgery went quite well. I believe the homeopath I chose did find the correct medicine for me. The whole experience really made me reexamine my values and has led to our moving to a smaller home on an island in a community-oriented, rural setting. I try to remind myself not to work so hard, although it seems to be my nature to do too much. My recent mammogram was quite normal and I count my blessings every day.

 ## Description

Breast cancer is an abnormal, undifferentiated, and out-of-control growth of cells in the breast. One in every 8 or 9 women in the United States will develop breast cancer, although the actual risk is only 1 in 2,500 at age twenty, 1 in 63 at age forty, 1 in 28 at age sixty, and 1 in 8 at age ninety. Breast cancer is the number one cause of cancer death in women in this country in women aged forty to forty-five; however, heart disease does kill six times more women than breast cancer.[1] Approximately 1 out of 4 women with breast cancer dies of it.

The degree and extent of the breast cancer varies tremendously. The main risk factors seem to be a family history; a high intake of fat, alcohol, and sugar; early menarche; late menopause; lack of pregnancies or late first pregnancy; or excess estrogen. This said, many women with an overall low risk for breast cancer do find themselves inexplicably diagnosed with the disease.

Symptoms

Four out of five women discover breast cancer themselves in the form of a lump found during a breast self-examination. Less often there is pain, cyclic breast cysts, discharge, inflammation, lumps in the armpit, or other visible changes in the breast such as discoloration or pulling. In many cases, such as with ductal carcinoma in situ (DCIS), you may have no symptoms and the condition may be discovered on a routine mammogram. If you suspect that you might have DCIS, request a magnified mammogram. This is the only way my DCIS was found; it was confirmed by a stereotactic biopsy.

Complications

Disfigurement due to lumpectomy or mastectomy can be a problem, but the most severe consequence of breast cancer is prolonged deterioration, suffering, and loss of life.

Conventional Treatment

The recommended treatment varies greatly with the type and extent of cancer and ranges from lumpectomy to mastectomy, radiation, chemotherapy, and bone marrow or stem cell transplants.

What to Expect from Homeopathic Treatment

Although the homeopathic literature documents cured cases of breast cancer, particularly in India, the medico-legal situation in this country, the potentially severe risks of depending on only one therapy, and the availability of numerous studies corroborating the effectiveness of other therapies, both conventional and alternative, makes it unwise to rely on homeopathy alone. I have treated over twenty-five women who used homeopathy as an adjunct to their conventional treatment with considerable success.

Most of my breast cancer patients have rebounded quickly from surgery and have had fewer and more manageable side effects from radiation and chemotherapy. Naturopathic and homeopathic treatment has provided hope, encouragement, and healing. I have been able to help them educate themselves, sort through their options for conventional treatment, and provide suggestions on positive attitude, empowerment, and spiritual connection.

Naturopathic Suggestions to Complement Homeopathic Care

• Eat a low-fat, vegetarian or primarily vegetarian diet with lots of fiber, legumes, and fresh fruits and vegetables.
• Buy organic produce. If you can't, then wash the produce with one of the commercial products that removes pesticide and chemical residues.
• If you choose to eat poultry, limit it and stick to free-range, hormone- and antibiotic-free brands.
• If you are a fish-eater, salmon, cod, and herring are recommended.
• Fish oil capsules can supplement your omega-3 fatty acids.
• Use olive oil rather than saturated fats.
• You'd be wise to avoid, or at least minimize, dairy products.
• Minimize or eliminate alcohol, caffeine, and sugar.
• Eat lots of soy (realize that there is some controversy about this and do your homework) and flax.
• Drink at least six glasses of water a day.
• Lipotropic factors, particularly in combination with liver herbs such as dandelion root and milk thistle, can help the liver break down estrogen.
• Do not smoke.
• Get rid of your underwire bras.
• Increase your intake of cabbage-family vegetables (including broccoli, cauliflower, cabbage, Brussels sprouts, rutabagas, bok choy, and kale).
• If you have had breast cancer, hormone-replacement therapy is not advised.
• Take a high-quality megamultivitamin and mineral, including vitamin E, 400 to 800 IU; and vitamin D, 400 to 1,000 IU; daily.
• Take 300 milligrams a day of Coenzyme Q_{10}.

- Ashwagandha is an Ayurvedic herb with tumor-reducing properties that I include in my daily regimen.
- Drink lots of green tea (decaffeinated is available), or take green tea supplements (one capsule can be equivalent to two or three cups).
- Decrease stress and do what you love.

Cervical Dysplasia
(See Genital Warts)

Depression

Lisa's Story

"I turned forty the year that I finally made an appointment for myself with Judyth. After I had made sure that she treated the rest of my family, all four children and my husband, then I could take my turn. As a mom, I felt it was my duty to get everybody else the help they needed first. Three of my four children had been diagnosed with ADHD (attention-deficit/hyperactivity disorder) and my husband had relied on antidepressants for several years. But when all of the 'fixing' of the rest of my family didn't 'fix' me, I realized I needed help, too.

"For most of my life, I was convinced there was a 'black hole' in my heart that nothing could fill. I had suffered intense loneliness most of my life, even though I was surrounded by family and friends. Nothing and no one ever filled it.

"I gave birth to my first baby when I was twenty-three. After a completely uneventful pregnancy, all of a sudden I started crying the very next day and didn't stop for the next twenty-one years! Five miscarriages followed over the course of the next five years. I bounced up and down on such a hormonal roller coaster than I couldn't even watch Pampers commercials without bawling. Finally, after being told that I could never give birth to any more children, we adopted a son. I believed he would fill the hole in my heart, but he didn't.

"The intense loneliness and crying jags just went on and on. Then I discovered I was pregnant again and, contrary to what my doctor had told me, my pregnancy was successful. The next five years brought two more miscarriages. My depression grew more and more intense. My spontaneity flew out the window. I insisted that everything be planned and regimented. Not only was I totally unable to enjoy life, but I took all the fun out of it for everybody around me. When friends dropped by unexpectedly to invite us to take a drive through a gorgeous canyon to admire the autumn leaves, I crumpled in a corner and cried.

"My periods had been irregular and painful since they began when I was twelve. They would come every six to eight weeks, and the cramps were so incapacitating that they kept me in bed for at least half a day each month.

"The homeopathic medicine that Judyth gave me at the end of that first appointment five years ago literally changed my life. My crying jags are nonexistent. I feel happier than I have since high school and am again able to enjoy my life. My periods are regular and there is minimal, if any, cramping. Homeopathy not only changed my life, but I honestly feel that it saved my family."

Lisa was a straight-from-the-book picture of *Pulsatilla* (windflower): soft, sensitive, weepy, changeable, and she put everyone else first. *Pulsatilla* is the only medicine she has needed since she began homeopathic treatment three years ago, except for a couple of doses of *Silica* (flint, a complementary medicine to *Pulsatilla*) for an ingrown toenail. If you have seen this plant, also called anemone, you will notice that it comes in an array of lovely colors like purple and pink, with a black center, and is very attractive. Lisa has the knack of looking like a million dollars, even though she shops at thrift stores—she looks like a flower in full bloom.

Women needing *Pulsatilla* typically have lots of hormonal problems, beginning with irregular and/or painful periods, then heavy bleeding, and often PMS and tend to feel the best in their lives when they are pregnant.

The feeling of having a black hole inside, along with Lisa's tendency to cry easily, her PMS, her desire to please, and her soft, warm, caring nature fit *Pulsatilla* very well. Lisa's menstrual flow is much lighter, her cramps substantially less, and her fuse is a lot longer. Her heartburn has improved so much that she has forgotten that she ever had it. Compared to her energy level before homeopathy, Lisa's energy is very good and she is a lot happier.

Marie's Story

"Homeopathy changed my life. It may even have saved it. I started seeing Judyth about nine years ago when I was depressed and confused. At that time I had also been taking an anti-seizure medication for fifteen years.

"There was a time when I thought I was losing it. I was bewildered, upset, and desperate enough to contemplate suicide. This was tough because throughout my career I have held positions of responsibility, positions that require me to be clear and on top of things. I generally know my mind and rarely feel confused. But once, while shopping for colored pencils, I simply couldn't figure out which colors I already had and which ones I needed. In the process of sorting this out at the art store, I lost thirty minutes while trying to make a decision about one little pencil! It was clear that something was wrong. When I explained it to Judyth, she took it as a clue and gave me a homeopathic medicine that solved the problem, along with a number of others.

"I tend to notice mental and emotional cues before physical ones. For example, I sometimes have thoughts of car crashes. I used to think this was just a coincidence or that I was being weird. Just driving along and imagining my car crashing into oncoming traffic or veering off the road. For Judyth, that thought was a clear confirmation of a homeopathic medicine. Over the years, I've learned how to pay attention to thoughts like this and report them at our appointments so they can lead to selecting the right medicine for me. I used to be afraid of such thoughts and wanted them to go away. Now I know they are a sign that I need something and I know how to get help.

"Getting rid of my seizure medication took a while, but today I am seizure-free and have been off the drugs for three years. I rarely feel depressed and when I begin to experience the confusion, I know it means I need another dose of my medicine.

"I also use homeopathy to treat acute conditions at home. The first place I look to for help is homeopathy. I go to an allopathic medical doctor for annual exams. For everything else I rely on homeopathy."

I have seen Marie for ten years for a wide variety of problems, including depression, fatigue, seizures, joint pain, constipation, weight problems, swelling of the salivary gland, upper respiratory infections, hypothyroidism, genital warts, urinary tract infection, vaginitis, ovarian pain, and a neuroma. Over the years, the medicines that have most helped Marie are *Silica* (flint), *Calcarea carbonica* (calcium carbonate), and *Aurum metallicum* (gold).

The most clearly differentiating feature of Marie's case recently has been a combination of grief over losing her mother and an exaggerated feeling of responsibility toward her dying mother and her colleagues at work. Just after the death of her mother, Marie suffered from bronchitis, during which time her mental state again slipped. She felt ready to give up and felt stuck in a deep, dark, black hole. Even though her acute illness was not even serious, much less life threatening, the toll of the grief and excessive responsibility pushed her over the edge. Marie felt as if she couldn't possibly get well, could not possibly miss even one more day of work after having taken time off to care for her mother, and could not let anyone else down. A dose of *Aurum metallicum* totally pulled her out of this dark state. She called the next day to tell me she felt so much better.

I always look forward to seeing Marie. Every one of her problems has responded positively to homeopathic treatment and she has even lost fifty pounds over the past two years though a disciplined program of diet and exercise.

Description

Depression ranges from a mild feeling of discontentment to an overwhelming feeling of sadness, hopelessness, and despair. You, as a woman, are much more likely to recognize and seek treatment for depression than are your male counterparts. Depression can become considerably worse with hormonal fluctuations such as periods, pregnancy, miscarriages, and menopause.

Symptoms

Mental and emotional symptoms include despair, loss of interest in life, emptiness, anxiety, irritability, desire to isolate yourself, confusion, impaired memory, and generally feeling overwhelmed. Physical symptoms such as fatigue, change in appetite and sleep, and weight loss or gain are also common.

Complications

The most common complications of depression are incapacity (due to severe depression) to lead your normal life and the devastating effect depression can have on other family members. The most severe outcome of depression, of course, is suicide.

Conventional Treatment

Antidepressants are widely prescribed, especially the SSRIs (selective serotonin reuptake inhibitors) such as Prozac. Other medications may be prescribed for sleep problems, anxiety, and the other components that accompany the depression.

What to Expect from Homeopathic Treatment

Depression and its accompanying symptoms generally respond very well to homeopathic treatment, whether or not the cause is related to hormones or something else and regardless of whether the depression is recent or lifelong. I have treated many women successfully for severe as well as mild depression, and for a variety of other psychiatric conditions such as mood swings, bipolar disorder, anxiety, phobias, panic attacks, obsessive-compulsive disorder, and even multiple personality disorder (now called dissociative identity disorder) and schizophrenia. To read about the many people my husband and I have successfully treated for these problems, refer to our book *Prozac-Free: Homeopathic Medicine for Depression, Anxiety and Other Mental and Emotional Problems.*

Naturopathic Suggestions to Complement Homeopathic Care

- Eat a healthful, balanced diet that is high in whole grains, fruits, vegetables, and fiber.
- If you tend toward hypoglycemia, be sure you eat plenty of protein; limit concentrated sources of simple carbohydrates such as juice, dried fruits, and sweets; and don't go too long without eating.
- Drink at least six glasses of water a day.
- Many women find St. John's wort, 300 milligrams three times a day, to lift their spirits, although this is not usually necessary if one is under homeopathic treatment.
- If you feel anxiety along with your depression, herbs such as passionflower, valerian, skullcap, hops, and chamomile can be quite soothing. SAMe can be useful for depression as well as arthritis.
- Make every effort to be in the present moment rather than obsessing about your past mistakes or losses or what may or may not ever happen in the future.
- Take one day at a time and put your energy into what is most important in your life and what you really can change, and let the rest go.
- Worry and guilt don't make anything better and can take quite a toll on your energy and peace of mind.
- If you are depressed, stay busy. I'm not suggesting that you ignore your problem. Do get whatever help you need, but don't spend all of your time dwelling on your unhappiness.
- Some excellent short-term psychotherapy techniques, such as rapid eye movement, thought field therapy, NLP (neurolinguistic programming), and Ericksonian hypnosis, can be great aids to stabilizing your moods.
- Surround yourself with people and pets that love and care about you and will support you when you need it.
- Exercise aerobically on a regular basis.
- Soaking up the wonder and beauty of nature is a super antidepressant.

DEPRESSION

- Yoga, meditation, contemplation, and prayer can elevate your mood tremendously.

Eating Disorders

Sally's Story

"As a child I was raised in a very dysfunctional family. My parents fought often at the dinner table. This affected my eating habits greatly. Since I was a young girl, I have struggled with an eating disorder. My mother, not knowing what to do with me, considered putting me in the hospital. As a teenager I went through counseling and various antidepressants. Nothing seemed to work in the long run. Nothing seemed to help me live a "normal" life. I felt isolated, confused, anxious, depressed, frustrated, out of control, and ashamed. I was a professional woman who, on the outside, seemed to have everything. The medications the doctors had me on seemed to work for about one year and then my symptoms would return. They would increase my dosage, which only increased the side effects. Any change in my routine would set me on a hidden path of chaos.

"Out of desperation, I did some research about homeopathy and thought that maybe it could help me. After attending a weekend seminar, I made an appointment with Dr. Reichenberg-Ullman. She and I worked together as a team, looking at all my symptoms—not just the eating disorder, but what was underlying it. The first session felt a bit odd, and I wondered why she asked me specific questions that pertained to my physical, mental, and emotional states. Conventional doctors did not take the time to really ask me about myself and just sit and listen, only offering me guidance.

"For a year and a half Dr. Reichenberg-Ullman worked with me to eliminate my immediate symptoms, slowly progressing to the real issue of my eating disorder. During the catharsis, my remedy changed and some of my symptoms got worse, but we kept working together. Since I've been on my remedy, I feel in control of my life; and although crises have hit I have been able to ride through them with a sense of control. I am much more in touch with my body. I can sense when I'm in need of my remedy.

"Homeopathy has benefited me long-term by alleviating my symptoms and providing me with a sense of physical, mental, and emotional balance—something I was unable to ever feel before."

I first saw Sally as a patient five years ago when she was twenty-eight. At the age of twelve, she began to throw up whenever she ate or else she wouldn't eat at all, pretending to forget that she was hungry. After months of fainting every morning in her English class, her teacher finally figured out she needed food. Sally was butting heads with her stepmother at the time. Later on, she only threw up after eating fattening food or after arguing, which reminded her of her parents' bickering when she was little. She found it impossible to eat in the school cafeteria amidst a din of loud voices. Yearning for a Barbie-doll figure, she roller-skated like crazy. As she grew older, she did not ever feel quite like she fit in. A high achiever, Sally was always working on improving herself in one way or another.

In addition, Sally's periods were irregular and very heavy, and her cramping was severe. She developed vaginitis, chlamydia, and carcinoma of the cervix, from which she fortunately recovered. She also complained of gas, bloating, PMS, anxiety attacks, and headaches.

The two medicines that have been most helpful for Sally were *Vanadium,* an excellent medicine for women whose happiness depends on their degree of success or failure and who tend toward anorexia and bulimia, and *Carcinosin* (nosode), because of her perfectionism and fastidiousness. She's not nearly as hard on herself now, her physical symptoms are considerably improved across the board, her eating is much more normal, she is in a terrific relationship, and she is pursuing a career she's really excited about.

Description

Anorexia nervosa (significant weight loss due to a distorted sense of body image and exaggerated fear of obesity, often accompanied by cessation of menstrual periods), bulimia (binge eating followed by self-induced vomiting and/or the use of laxatives and diuretics), and obesity (greater than 20 percent over normal weight) are the three main manifestations of eating disorders. Anorexia and bulimia are considered by conventional medicine to be psychiatric problems, while obesity, despite the fact that psychological factors do often come into play, is not. These eating patterns may allow eating huge amounts of food, such as an entire cake or a quart of ice cream, at one sitting followed by vomiting or using some means of purging. Extreme exercise routines are often part of the picture.

Symptoms

Symptoms, which may be overt or hidden, can include marked weight loss, an overconcern with weight gain and eating high-calorie foods to the point of meticulously weighing or measuring foods, counting calories, and drastically reducing food intake. In the case of obesity, it is the weight gain that is exaggerated. Physical symptoms may include amenorrhea (lack of periods), low heart rate and blood pressure, coldness, and stomach and/or abdominal pain or discomfort.

Complications
Loss of periods, osteoporosis, and, in extreme cases, death can result from extended periods of anorexia.

Conventional Treatment
The three main interventions in orthodox medicine are antidepressants, psychotherapy, and, in severe or life-threatening situations, medical intervention requiring hospitalization.

What to Expect from Homeopathic Treatment
Homeopathic treatment can help turn around attitude and self-image, as well as depression and any other mental and emotional or physical complaints. You have to want help, though, and not be so deeply entrenched in your beliefs that you are unwilling to change.

Naturopathic Suggestions to Complement Homeopathic Care
• Explore the underlying cause of the eating disorder through whatever form of psychotherapy you choose.
• While you are doing some form of therapy, reduce the stress in your life, find friends and family in whom you can confide, and share your feelings rather than hide them.
• Specific dietary interventions are unlikely to work until you get to the root of the problem, but a healthful diet of whole grains, organic fruits and vegetables, fiber, and adequate protein is ideal.
• Drink at least six glasses of water a day to keep your body lubricated.
• If you have an eating disorder and tend to be thin and small-boned and have dry skin, nervousness, insomnia, and gas, Ayurvedic medicine would classify you as having a Vata constitution. The recommendation is to drink lots of liquids, preferably warm or hot; include olive and/or canola oil in your diet; rub your body with sesame oil on a regular basis; avoid or minimize foods that give you gas, such as the cabbage family and beans; choose cooked over raw vegetables; and relax. I know that oil is repulsive to many

women with eating disorders, but if this description fits you, it may be just what you need.

- Take a high-quality multivitamin and mineral with plenty of calcium and magnesium.
- If you do not have periods due to anorexia, herbs such as chaste tree and black cohosh, as well as natural progesterone cream (which contains wild yam), can be very helpful in bringing your periods back to normal.
- Aerobic exercise for twenty to thirty minutes a day, three to four times a week is adequate. You may be used to much more exercise than this as part of your self-imposed weight-loss program.
- Yoga not only stretches and tones the body, but it eases the mind and soothes the spirit.
- Nurture yourself with massages, time spent out in nature, and your favorite activities.

Endometriosis

Janine's Story

"I originally turned to homeopathy eight years ago for relief from terrible seasonal hay fever. I had tried basically every prescription drug available over a period of about ten years, with relatively little success. My homeopathic treatments not only gave me great relief from my allergies, but helped me in many other unexpected areas as well. The bladder and yeast infections that plagued me almost a dozen times a year vanished. My chronically dry skin and scalp were repaired. My periods were no longer accompanied by heavy bleeding and horrible cramps. In fact, most months, I no longer even had to take an aspirin for the pain.

"About two years after beginning homeopathy, I discovered that I had endometriosis and that it had probably been with me for a long time. I truly believe that homeopathy slowed the growth of the disease before it became debilitating or caused extensive damage to my reproductive organs. The evidence of this is the almost complete disappearance of severe menstrual cramping, which is often a result of endometriosis. Thanks to homeopathy, I was able to become pregnant with only a minimal amount of invasive procedures. My husband and I now have a beautiful baby girl to cherish and she has also benefited greatly from homeopathic treatment. Homeopathy has greatly improved the quality of my life!"

Homeopathy has been a gift for Janine in a number of ways. When I first saw her five years ago at the age of twenty-five, she was plagued by allergies. Her nose was perpetually congested, causing her to have sinus headaches three times a week. In addition, her frequent gas and belching; her dry, scaly skin and dandruff; and her discomfort with change all led me to prescribe *Lycopodium* (club moss). Another indication was the contrast between her shyness in a room full of strangers and her self-description as a loudmouth with people she knew well. All of these symptoms were improved by the homeopathy.

Two and a half years later, because of her strong need to have control over her life and "have her whole future planned out," her constant feeling of being wound up and high-strung, and her litany of what-ifs, as well as her fear of heights, her strong sweet tooth, and her overconcern about arriving at appointments on time, I changed the medicine to *Argentum nitricum* (silver nitrate). Janine still needs a dose occasionally, but she is quite happy and healthy overall. So is her delightful little girl, Sophie, who is worlds more fun to be around since she was given *Chamomilla* (chamomile) for her temper tantrums.

Description

Endometriosis is the presence of endometrial tissue (from the uterus) in places where it should not normally be. The condition is found in 10 to 15 percent of women between twenty-five and forty-four who are menstruating.

Symptoms

You may experience no symptoms whatsoever. Or you might have pain that varies from slight to incapacitating and in areas all the way from your rectum to your lungs, depending on the site(s) of the outgrowth. Pain is often worse premenstrually, around your period, or during sex. Bowel or bladder problems may arise, depending on the location of the endometriosis, though pelvic pain is far more common. The only sure way to diagnose endometriosis is through laparoscopy, a surgical procedure.

Complications

The most frequent complication is infertility.

Conventional Treatment

Hormones are the treatment of choice for conventional doctors. These may be in the form of birth control pills, synthetic progestin, Danazol, and drugs such as Lupron and Synarel. The next route is surgery, which is often used in combination with hormones, in which the endometrial tissue is removed. The last resort is a hysterectomy. Orthodox medicine, in my opinion, still has quite a barbaric approach to treating endometriosis. The endometrial tissue often grows back within months of surgery and some of the hormones throw a woman, temporarily, into a premature menopausal state or have side effects that are even worse than the endometriosis. Many women go back and forth between various courses of hormones and surgeries without significant benefit.

What to Expect from Homeopathic Treatment

Given the conventional alternatives, I would strongly urge any woman with endometriosis to give homeopathy a year or two before resorting to more invasive and traumatic modes of therapy.

Naturopathic Suggestions to Complement Homeopathic Care

- Reduce your intake of animal products, including dairy.
- Eat a diet high in whole grains, fresh fruits and vegetables, and fiber.
- Drink at least six glasses of water a day.
- Lipotropic factors, particularly in combination with liver herbs such as dandelion root and milk thistle, can help the liver break down estrogen.
- Eliminate caffeine, sugar, and alcohol.
- Eat salmon, mackerel, and cod, or take fish oil capsules.
- Eat 1 tablespoon of ground flaxseeds a day or 1 tablespoon of flaxseed oil.
- Take evening primrose, black currant, or borage oil.
- Some women find natural progesterone cream helpful.
- Investigate and resolve any psychological issues that might be exacerbating the problem.

Fibrocystic Breasts

Sarah's Story

"Cancer in the family is certainly a motivating factor for change! My younger sister died of breast cancer at thirty-one. That same year biopsy results showed that I had atypical breast tissue that put me at a very high risk for developing breast cancer myself. 'Two options,' warned the surgeon. 'Tamoxifen or cut off your breasts.' Neither seemed terribly appealing, so I decided to seek out another alternative and found Judyth.

"I was drinking way too much coffee at the time. Judyth explained that my body was not breaking down estrogen sufficiently and encouraged me to change my diet completely. I embarked on a vegan (nondairy vegetarian) diet with fish, as well as taking a number of supplements that included a megamultivitamin and mineral, an herbal formula to help the liver break down estrogen, soy isolate, and a few others. She also treated me with a homeopathic medicine that eliminated my continual breast soreness.

"I'm not sure how and why it all works, but I'm delighted with the whole program. My mammograms have shown no further development of atypical cells since I started seeing Judyth seven years ago and I am healthy."

Along with eliminating caffeine and making the other suggested dietary changes, Sarah relieved her breast pain by taking *Conium* (hemlock). It is an excellent medicine for breast lumps, especially if they are hard, as well as for uterine fibroids. It can be useful for women whose sexual outlets have been prematurely cut off, such as after the death of a partner. Over the more than seven years that I have treated Sarah, she has gone on to need other homeopathic medicines for a variety of complaints.

Description
Fibrocystic breast disease (FBD) can cause heaviness, swelling, discomfort, or pain of the breasts, usually sometime between ovulation and the onset of your period.

Symptoms
Symptoms range from a slight but tolerable swelling and discomfort to pain so intense that putting on a bra, exercise, or even movement is terribly painful.

Complications
Although fibrocystic breast disease is in itself quite benign, an increase in cystic tissue in the breast can sometimes, as happened to me, be a forewarning of more serious changes in the breast tissue.

Conventional Treatment

Using birth control pills, taking synthetic progesterone, and eliminating caffeine are the most common recommendations.

What to Expect from Homeopathic Treatment

Homeopathy can be of great benefit for fibrocystic breasts, particularly if supplemented by a few dietary and nutritional changes.

Naturopathic Suggestions to Complement Homeopathic Care

- Eat a diet high in whole grains, fruits, vegetables, and fiber with adequate protein (and limited animal products).
- Drink at least six glasses of water a day.
- Eliminate all sources of caffeine completely, including chocolate.
- Take vitamin E, 400 to 800 IU a day.
- Make sure your dietary fat does not contribute more than 20 percent of your daily caloric intake.
- Take evening primrose, black currant, or borage oil.
- Increase your iodine intake through seafood and sea vegetables.
- You may find natural progesterone cream to be helpful.

Gallstones

Nan's Story

"Two years ago I began to develop intense pain just below my right rib cage that radiated to my right shoulder blade. It seemed to come on after I ate rich foods, which, of course, I love. Judyth had already helped me tremendously with my arthritis, and homeopathy seemed highly preferable to having my gallbladder taken out!

"I was given a medicine to keep on hand when I felt my gallbladder symptoms coming on. Any time there is even a hint of my symptoms, I reach for it and the pain is relieved almost immediately. It's a miracle!"

Nan's main problems over the past four years, since she first came to see me, have been joint stiffness and gallbladder pain. *Rhus toxicodendron* (poison ivy) given a few times a year has consistently taken care of her musculoskeletal complaints. I have prescribed five doses of *Chelidonium* (Greater celantine) during the past two years for Nan when she has experienced intense, severe pain radiating from her gallbladder area to her shoulder blades, accompanied by lots of burping and a preference for hot water. Each time Nan has taken the *Chelidonium* (after eating foods that are admittedly too rich for her system), all of her symptoms have gone away quickly.

Description
Pain is usually due to an acute inflammation of the wall of your gallbladder, generally as a result of an obstruction of the duct by a gallstone.

Symptoms
Pain in the area of the gallbladder (just under the right rib cage) generally progresses from colic to severe pain and often radiates to the lower part of the right shoulder blade. It is often recurrent. Nausea and vomiting are quite common, as well as a low-grade fever.

Complications
Most of the time gallbladder pain becomes so acute that some type of care, often in the form of a visit to the emergency room, is required. However, if the condition progresses untreated, obstructive jaundice can occur.

Conventional Treatment
Antibiotics, intravenous fluids and electrolytes, and removal of the gallbladder are the typical protocol.

What to Expect from Homeopathic Treatment
Homeopathy can keep the symptoms at bay, as you can see from the previous case, and prevent surgery, especially if rich foods are avoided or kept to a minimum. If the gallbladder bursts, peritonitis, which may be fatal, can occur.

Naturopathic Suggestions to Complement Homeopathic Care
- Eat a diet high in whole grains, organic, fresh fruits and vegetables, and adequate protein.
- Drink at least six glasses of water a day.
- Reduce your intake of fatty and rich foods.
- Eat a high-fiber diet.

- Increase your intake of vegetables and soy.
- Take lipotropic factors to remove fat deposits from the liver.
- Liver herbs such as dandelion root and milk thistle can be helpful but are usually not necessary if you are being treated homeopathically.
- Castor oil packs over the gallbladder may help acute pain.

Genital Warts (Human Papilloma Virus) and Cervical Dysplasia

Jamie's Story

"Some specific conditions homeopathy has really helped me with are vaginal yeast infections, urinary tract infections, and genital warts, as well as eczema, colds, the flu, bronchitis, and depression. I've especially appreciated the simple and easy remedies for vaginal infections. My gynecologist prescribed Monistat-7, but Judyth recommended lactobacillus and boric acid suppositories that solved the problem for me.

"A routine Pap smear showed that I had genital warts caused by HPV, a virus that can result in cervical cancer. I was extremely upset. The only option I was offered to get rid of the warts was to freeze them and cut them off. Yikes! Being a patient of homeopathic medicine for so long, I knew that this wasn't the answer. It only addressed the symptom and not the cause. I went to Judyth and she gave me a homeopathic medicine. Within a few weeks the external warts went away. My next visit to the gynecologist produced a normal Pap smear. Now, two years later, some of the warts have returned, but I am confident that with homeopathic medicine, this will be something I can keep under control without invasive procedures.

"I could tell many stories about how homeopathy has helped me. Mostly, I would like to say how grateful I am to have a doctor who truly listens and hears what I have to tell her. And that I have discovered a form of medicine that I can feel truly good about taking and am assured that the side effects won't be worse than the symptoms. I know that I'm doing something really good for my health now, when I'm young, and probably preventing more serious diseases and problems that come from continually suppressing what's wrong. Homeopathy works!"

Jamie is an introspective, deep-thinking, mature young woman who has been sensitive to the emotional wounds of disappointed love. Quite affected by music and preferring to keep her tears to herself, she fits the picture of *Natrum muriaticum* (sodium chloride) quite nicely and it has been the only medicine she has needed over six and a half years, with the exception of one dose of *Thuja* (arbor vitae), which resulted in the disappearance of her genital warts the first time. All of her other physical symptoms, including sinus headaches, dandruff, urinary tract infections, bronchitis, and Raynaud's syndrome, have responded to the *Natrum muriaticum*. It alleviated her depression and anxiety attacks as well.

Description

Cervical dysplasia is a progressive pattern of abnormal cell changes in the cervix, based on the results of a Pap smear. Changes may vary from slight, due to inflammation or infection, all the way to cervical cancer. About 90 percent of cervical dysplasia can be attributed to human papilloma virus (HPV)[2]. At least half of the normal adult population in the United States and 40 percent of children are estimated to show evidence of HPV infection; however, most women exposed to HPV do *not* develop either genital warts or cervical dysplasia.[3] Fortunately, the alteration in cells tends to be quite gradual and can generally be caught early. The two women who have come to me with cervical cancer had gone five and ten years without getting a Pap smear. Cervical cancer is preventable. Please make sure you go to your women's health-care specialist for regular Pap smears.

Symptoms

Cervical dysplasia is often asymptomatic and only detectable through a screening Pap smear, followed, if appropriate, by a colposcopy and biopsy. Women with HPV often have warts on the outside of the vulva, but they can just as easily be located only in the vagina or on the cervix.

Complications

The greatest complication is cervical cancer, which can end up necessitating a hysterectomy, and can ultimately result in death.

Conventional Treatment

The main conventional treatments for genital warts are laser surgery, topical Podophyllin or acid, cryocautery (freezing), and electrocautery (including the loop electrode excision procedure, or LEEP). None of these methods is considered curative. The warts are removed, but the underlying cause is not addressed.

What to Expect from Homeopathic Treatment

I have found a combination of homeopathy and the other interventions mentioned further on to be effective in normalizing Pap smears in all but one patient I have treated. The one exception was a woman who did not deal with the underlying psychological reasons that made her susceptible to recurrent episodes of dysplasia. I have had mixed results in eliminating venereal warts; however, even in those cases where some warts remain, the Pap smears have been otherwise normal, and the women have felt better in all other ways.

Naturopathic Suggestions to Complement Homeopathic Care

- Eat a diet high in whole grains, fruits, vegetables, and fiber with adequate protein (and limited in animal products).
- Drink at least six glasses of water a day.
- Eliminate all sources of caffeine completely, including chocolate.
- Have Pap smears and pelvic exams every year.
- Do a regular self-examination of your genital area.
- Do not smoke.
- Be discriminating about your sexual partners.
- Use condoms.
- If you take birth control pills, which in most cases I do not advise, supplement with folic acid (which they deplete).
- Take folic acid, 5 milligrams two times a day orally, and mixed carotenes, 150,000 IU a day for three months, then repeat your Pap smear. I recommend doing this under the guidance of a naturopathic physician, who can use additional interventions if necessary.
- Do whatever inner work is needed to remove any psychological blocks to healing your cervix, such as dealing with past sexual abuse, unhappy intimate relationships, or lack of self-love.

Headaches (Hormonally Caused)

Debbie's Story

"Before I found Dr. Reichenberg-Ullman eight years ago, my periods disrupted my life because of severe pain, very heavy bleeding that included passing huge clots, and significantly disturbing PMS mood swings. I also suffered from migraine headaches, which usually began the day before my period and were so debilitating that I had to stay in bed until they subsided.

"After receiving my homeopathic medicine, for the first time in years I didn't have to go to bed with a migraine, and the bleeding and pain diminished. Each month brought more relief, with symptoms returning only when I antidoted my medicine somehow. Another dose always put me back on track."

Debbie's headaches were excruciating and extreme. The head pain had started when she was in her twenties. When she became pregnant, after ten years of infertility, her headaches went away, only to return after she had nursed her baby for three and a half months. They occurred before, during, and after her periods and lasted a total of two weeks out of every month.

When Debbie first consulted me in November of 1991, she had just suffered six severe headaches the month before, each lasting one to two days. Along with the headaches came disorientation, irritability, inability to focus, and a feeling of disconnectedness, as if everything were moving in slow motion.

Debbie managed the pain with 1,000 milligrams of Tylenol every three to four hours. Light, even a small amount of noise, and any chaos or commotion were too much during her headaches. One headache was so unbearable that Debbie vomited for five days straight, even after taking sips of water.

Debbie also had a number of other symptoms, including mood swings, lots of moles, and a strong family history of cancer. The medicine that covers all of these symptoms, in addition to her maddening headaches, was *Carcinosin* (nosode). Two doses over a one-year period took away the headaches and mood swings and left her feeling so good that she has not needed further treatment. Her severe headaches have never returned.

HEADACHES
(Hormonally Caused)

Description
Headaches that are clearly associated with your periods, pregnancy, menopause, or taking birth control pills.

Symptoms
The intensity of pain varies tremendously, as with headaches in general, as do the frequency, duration, and degree of limitation of your normal activities.

Complications

The most severe complication is a brain tumor or aneurysm, but women with hormonally-induced headaches often report having them since the onset of their periods.

Conventional Treatment

Vasodilators and pain medications.

What to Expect from Homeopathic Treatment

Homeopathy has very good results in eliminating or greatly minimizing hormonal headaches.

Naturopathic Suggestions to Complement Homeopathic Care

- Eat a diet high in whole grains, fruits, vegetables, and fiber, with adequate protein (and limited in animal products).
- Drink at least six glasses of water a day.
- Eliminate all sources of caffeine completely, including chocolate.
- If there are other specific foods or drinks, such as wine, that trigger or worsen your headaches, avoid them.
- For congestive-type headaches, such as migraines, wrap a cold, wet cloth around your head or use an ice pack on your head while immersing your hands and feet in hot water.
- Lie down in a dark, quiet place where you will be undisturbed.
- Do long, deep, slow breathing as you imagine or visualize the pain being released.
- For tension headaches, soak in an Epsom salts tub.
- Press deeply on the two points just below the flat bone at the back of the skull, about two inches to either side of the center. This is good for tension headaches. Release when the pain diminishes or goes away.
- Massage your scalp and the trigger points along your neck and shoulders.
- Do whatever you can to de-stress to relieve your distress.

Heavy Periods
(See Menstrual Problems)

Herpes

Karen's Story

"I've had Type I herpes (cold sores) since I was a small child. My mother had them, so my guess is that she passed them on to me, and I was susceptible to them as well. Over the years I learned what worked and what didn't for my herpes, but basically they came, ran their course, and took a long time to go away. The only kind of medicine I used was over-the-counter.

"I started homeopathy about nine years ago, though not specifically for herpes, but for all of me. For the past few years, *Sepia* helped keep the outbreaks to a minimum and they were less severe. I only got an episode once or twice a year, and usually not a very bad case.

"Stress, diet, and lack of proper rest all affect whether or not I will get an outbreak. So I know to pay attention to these things, as well as to use homeopathy. In 1999 I had only one outbreak, and one was after a week-long seminar during which time I was exposed on a daily basis to lots of essential oils that antidoted my homeopathic medicine, as well as having too much exposure to the cold and wind and definitely not enough sleep. Homeopathy has helped keep the outbreaks small, few, and far between, and they are usually gone in a little over a week.

"I also contracted genital herpes in the late 1970s or early 1980s. My outbreaks have always been limited to one area. The last time I had an outbreak was at least six years ago."

When she first came to see me nine years ago, Karen suffered from major self-reproach and depression, as well as premenstrual rage and herpes. She was down all the time, especially during holidays—moody, sullen, and easy to anger. Though Karen realized she was unreasonably and impossibly hard on herself, she couldn't seem to let up. Karen's oral herpes began when she was a little girl and the genital herpes, ten years before our first visit. *Sepia* (cuttlefish ink) helped Karen reduce the frequency and intensity of her herpes outbreaks, both oral and genital. Her PMS improved substantially, as did her episodes of rage and her ability to appreciate herself. Whereas she felt stuck in many ways before the *Sepia* (which can be characteristic of women needing it), since taking it she has bought her own home and is much happier with her job. Karen is unreasonably demanding of herself but is learning to recognize at least some of her many positive qualities. Over the past couple of years, the homeopathic medicine *Chocolate* has helped Karen to feel even better.

Description

Ulcers on the lips (cold sores or fever blisters, Type I) or an infection of the genitals and around the rectum associated (Type II) with the herpes simplex II virus.

Symptoms

The lesions in either place tend to occur as clusters of small, blister-like eruptions that crust over after a few days and usually heal in about ten days. If genital, they may occur on the labia, clitoris, vagina, cervix, or perineum. In addition to the numbness, tingling, itching, and soreness of the eruptions, the first outbreak is often accompanied by flulike symptoms, including fever, fatigue, and difficult urination.

Complications

Though genital herpes may be accompanied, rarely, by other neurological diseases, the main complication for women is transmission to the newborn child during pregnancy. An active lesion at the time of delivery often necessitates a cesarean section.

Conventional Treatment

Topical analgesics and PABA are the most common treatments for oral herpes. Acyclovir, available in oral, topical, and intravenous forms, is the treatment of choice in conventional medicine.

What to Expect from Homeopathic Treatment

Homeopathy is generally very effective in decreasing the frequency and intensity of outbreaks to the point where they are not a problem. I have found that a predisposition to oral herpes generally means an increased susceptibility to genital herpes, although sexual transmission must occur in some form for Type II to occur.

Naturopathic Suggestions to Complement Homeopathic Care

• Eat a diet high in lysine-containing foods (vegetables, fish, chicken, turkey, beans, cashews, and brewer's yeast) and low in arginine-containing foods, such as chocolate, nuts, and seeds.
• Drink at least six glasses of water a day.

- Eliminate all sources of caffeine completely, including chocolate.
- Avoid any other substances or stressors that seem to trigger outbreaks for you.
- Take lysine, 1,000 milligrams a day, and triple the dose during an outbreak.
- Apply ice or licorice ointment or gel to lesions during an outbreak.
- Take vitamin C, 1,000 milligrams a day.
- Practice safe sex, be discriminating about your sexual partners, and use condoms.

Incontinence

Elise's Story

"At age fifty-four, when I first consulted Dr. Reichenberg-Ullman, I experienced a problem of awakening in the morning, or even sometimes in the middle of the night, with both hands asleep. Sometimes they would also go numb or feel like they were asleep while I held on to the steering wheel on long drives. I was also bothered by a progressive problem, at first annoying and then increasingly distressing, of stress incontinence. From the first dose of *Causticum,* both of these symptoms rapidly resolved. The improvement was, in fact, overnight. Over a period of ten years, a number of repetitions of the *Causticum* have been required, sometimes because of my having inadvertently antidoted the medicine and, after longer intervals, because of the spontaneous recurrence of symptoms. Each time, another dose of the *Causticum* has promptly corrected both problems."

One single homeopathic medicine has taken care of nearly all of Elise's problems, particularly her urinary incontinence, over the past ten years and that is *Causticum* (potassium hydrate). When I first saw her at age fifty-one, her main complaints were of stress incontinence on coughing or sneezing, occasional dribbling, uterine fibroids, a tickling cough with lots of throat clearing, numbness in the hands on waking after sleep, jaw pain, and metatarsal pain. All of Elise's problems were on the right side. A self-reliant and somewhat stoic woman, Elise was relatively fearless, enjoyed challenges, and didn't have anything to complain about other than her physical symptoms. Her anger would rarely flare up except when she felt someone was being mistreated, and she had always been drawn to helping learning disabled and handicapped children.

Elise has responded well with infrequent doses of the *Causticum* for these problems. She has straddled the fence between conventional medicine and homeopathy and did choose to have a hysterectomy for her fibroids and surgery for a breast tumor. I have found long-term homeopathic treatment to protect many women against serious illness, but this is, unfortunately, not always the case.

Description
Urinary incontinence is involuntary loss of urine.

Symptoms
Incontinence is characterized by dribbling, to a lesser or greater degree, most commonly when you cough, sneeze, or strain, or on exertion.

Complications
Incontinence is more of an annoyance and inconvenience than a serious condition.

Conventional Treatment
Mild cases may respond to Kegel's exercises. Otherwise, estriol cream, sympathomimetic (alpha-adrenergic) drugs, or even surgery are the conventional approaches.

What to Expect from Homeopathic Treatment
I would say that homeopathy has a reasonably good chance of improving or eliminating your incontinence.

Naturopathic Suggestions to Complement Homeopathic Care
- Do Kegel's exercises to strengthen the pubococcygeal muscle.
- Dr. Christiane Northrup reports good success with weighted cones placed in the vagina for a few minutes twice a day. I have no experience with this, but it sounds interesting. I refer you to her book, *Women's Bodies, Women's Wisdom.*
- Cut down on your intake of coffee and tea, both caffeinated and decaf.

- Urinate as soon as you feel the urge rather than putting it off until the time is right.
- Lose weight if you need to.
- Pessaries can help some women if surgery is not necessary.

Infertility

Kelly's Story

"The reason I was able to get pregnant is because I went to see Judyth. A year prior to starting homeopathy, I had a laparoscopy to surgically remove the endometrial tissue, but it came back within a few months. I refused to have yet another operation. I sought out alternative care, knowing somehow that there had to be a natural solution. I never dreamed that after my very first visit, I would no longer suffer from any of my symptoms and that I would be pregnant within three months!"

Kelly's infertility was due to endometriosis. She had also experienced a number of years of amenorrhea due to bulimia. Only three months after our first visit eight years ago, Kelly became pregnant after a number of years of trying futilely to do so. We were both thrilled. The medicine that helped her to do so was *Calcarea phosphorica* (calcium phosphate), prescribed because of her joint pain, terrible PMS since menarche, and a previous fracture that still flared up when it snowed.

Description

If you have tried to become pregnant unsuccessfully for one year without using any form of contraception, you fit the definition of infertility. Even women who have no hormonal problems can take a year or more to become pregnant.

Symptoms

If the infertility is due to problems with ovulation, polycystic ovaries, uterine fibroids, a previous chlamydial or gonorrheal infection, an endocrine imbalance, or a variety of other causes, there may be no symptoms at all other than the lack of becoming pregnant. If it is due to endometriosis, resulting in a blockage of a fallopian tube, you will probably experience pain with sex and painful periods, depending on the degree and location of the endometriosis.

Complications

None, other than the disappointment and heartbreak of not being able to conceive a child, except in the case of undiagnosed gonorrhea or syphilis, which can lead to joint and other more serious problems, or osteoporosis associated with prolonged amenorrhea (absence of periods).

Conventional Treatment

Treatment is highly variable, depending on the cause of the infertility.

What to Expect from Homeopathic Treatment

If the infertility is due to endometriosis, I have seen excellent results with homeopathy. If it is due to other factors, I have seen mixed results, but homeopathy is a lot safer and less invasive than conventional treatments and I recommend sticking with it for at least one year before looking to other interventions.

Naturopathic Suggestions to Complement Homeopathic Care

• Explore thoroughly the cause of your difficulty in conceiving. Make sure it is not due to your partner's low sperm count or other factors that have nothing to do with your own body.

• Know that great strides are being made in the treatment of infertility. Research each one carefully and follow the course of action that rings true to you and your partner, rather than what other people think is right for the two of you.

• There is no point in beating yourself up because you can't get pregnant. It may be that there are other plans ahead of you, such as adopting, foster-parenting, or reaching out in any number of ways to children who are not yours biologically.

• While you are trying to become pregnant, cultivate a positive attitude, trust that events will unfold as they need to, and remember that life is full of surprises.

• Live as healthful a lifestyle as possible, regardless of whether or not you bear a child.

• Take the opportunity to clear out any remaining baggage from your own childhood and heal any wounds between yourself and your parents.

Irregular Periods *(See Menstrual Problems)*

Low Sexual Energy

Bev's Story

"For several years after the birth of my first child, I felt tired. It was not just the tired you feel from long days with an active infant and then a busy toddler, but a deeper tiredness. My energy for most things was low. I felt sad and moody even though I had a wonderful, bright daughter. I sometimes just did not care. My sexual energy was nonexistent and I had periods of feeling blue. I thought I should be able to will myself through it. I just needed to try harder. I felt that postpartum depression should not still be the problem. Then I took *Sepia*. Slowly, over the next several weeks, I began to gain vitality. I enjoyed my family more and didn't feel so tired. My affection for my husband returned and, to our happiness, my second child was conceived."

Bev first came for help from homeopathy nine years ago at the age of thirty-five. She had a number of health problems, including constipation for five days at a time, heartburn, gas and bloating, and abdominal cramping. Her gynecological complaints included irregular periods since the age of eleven, uterine cramping and lower back pain, premenstrual irritability, and low sexual energy, especially since her first pregnancy. Bev was close to her husband but felt neutral sexually. She had experienced postpartum depression for over a year after the birth of her daughter, who was now five. She found herself crying more easily since her daughter was born, as well.

Bev derived great benefit from *Sepia* (cuttlefish ink), both before and after the birth of her next child. I gave her eight doses of *Sepia,* as needed, over a seven-year period. She has not needed the medicine for the past two years.

Description
This is a lack of sexual desire for any reason.

Symptoms
Your lack of or diminished sexual desire could be due to any number of reasons—physical (menopause, other hormonal or endocrine problems, fatigue, recent childbirth or nursing, etc.), mental/emotional (depression, interpersonal difficulties with your partner, history of sexual abuse, stress, trauma, or other factors), or just situational (too much work, the kids are always around, you're thinking too much about work). If there are actual

physical problems, you may experience associated symptoms; otherwise, you may be asymptomatic.

Complications
Disparity in sexual desire and energy is a frequent cause of relationship dissatisfaction.

Conventional Treatment
Treatment depends entirely on the cause of the decreased libido.

What to Expect from Homeopathic Treatment
Whether or not your libido will respond to homeopathy depends on numerous factors. There is certainly no guarantee, but it is definitely worth giving homeopathy a shot for a year. You may regain some, most, or all of your sexual energy, as did Bev, but even if your libido is not revived, the correct homeopathic medicine will alleviate most or all of your other symptoms and enhance your overall energy, clarity of thinking, health, and well-being.

Naturopathic Suggestions to Complement Homeopathic Care
• Explore any physiological causes for your diminished sex drive. The solution might be as simple as increasing your thyroid function or estrogen level.
• Find other ways to show love, affection, and deep caring for your partner.
• Go deeply within and ask yourself whether any internal obstruction stands in the way of a healthy sex life.
• Make sure you're eating and living in a healthful way, taking high-quality nutritional supplements, and getting lots of exercise and fresh air.
• Give it time. With menopause, for example, let your body, mind, and spirit ease into the transition before you start worrying too much about the change in your sexual energy.
• Herbs such as dong quai, vitex, and black cohosh can sometimes balance your hormones and bring back your sex drive.
• Progesterone cream is another way some women regain their libido.
• There are many other avenues to balance your life force and sexual energy, including yoga, Chi Gong, acupuncture, and Chinese herbs (may interfere with homeopathy), and other forms of energetic healing and bodywork.

Menopause

Elizabeth's Story

"I was first introduced to homeopathic medicine by an orthopedic doctor when I refused additional cortisone shots for bone pain. When I started menopause, I had already heard about a possible connection between estrogen replacement and cancer. I knew that the women in my family, including my mother and both grandmothers, had had breast cancer and I was unwilling to add any more risk to myself.

"I began to suffer from horrible hot flashes that woke me three to four times a night. I felt exhausted and could cry over anything. My right shoulder also bothered me on a regular basis. Dr. Bob [Ullman] punched my symptoms into his laptop and somehow came up with the right medicine and now I have neither hot flashes nor any other sign of menopause. My vitamins also help me keep up my energy.

"I had such doubts when we started homeopathic treatment. I did have to give up a few things, like permanents and coffee. I cheated at first, but soon realized how much better I felt without the coffee. It was well worth giving up. I can't believe how many women live with hot flashes just because they think they have to.

"Pay attention to your body. It speaks to you as long as you don't silence the conversation by taking drugs for every ache and pain. I don't take aspirin or sleep aids or cold medicines anymore. I increased my vitamin C and rest. I don't 'infect' my body with outside chemicals. There's no question in my mind now as to whether homeopathy works. My pain led me to try it. I don't understand why more women won't try a natural approach to health."

Dr. Ullman prescribed *Sanguinaria* (blood-root) for Elizabeth's hot flashes, frequent waking at night, grouchiness, and right shoulder stiffness. She has benefited from six doses of *Sanguinaria* over the past year and a half. Each time Elizabeth received the medicine, all of these symptoms greatly improved.

Some women, most often due to uterine fibroids or excessive menstrual bleeding and less frequently due to uterine or ovarian cancer, undergo a premature menopause. This was the case with Laurie, whom I began to see ten years ago.

Laurie's Story

"Homeopathy has not just been an alternative medicine for me. It has turned into a journey of long-term healing that has spanned ten years. When I first came to work with Judyth, I was a walking pharmacy, a hormonal nightmare, and a confused woman with a collection of physical and psychological ailments. I embarked on homeopathy at the ripe young age of thirty-five, about three years after I had a hysterectomy, including the removal of my ovaries. The story of how and why I had to have a hysterectomy is a separate one; however, it is accurate to say that if I had known about the positive effects of homeopathy before I had that irreversible operation, I would have explored that avenue first and perhaps spared myself the grief of having to deal with the overwhelming side effects that inevitably follow a hysterectomy.

"My status after the operation was awful, to put it mildly. My doctors reassured me that if I would faithfully take hormone replacements, then I would not suffer the symptoms of menopause. Wrong! My body just didn't conform the way they told me it would. I tried every method of hormone replacement known to woman, yet none of them could dispel my migraine headaches, hot flashes, swelling, and overall major depression that can accompany surgical menopause.

"In addition to all of the above, I was taking medication for an underfunctioning thyroid and for seizures. Add to that my having developed allergies to almost everything, from food to pollens and even to the replacement hormones! I felt overwhelmed and yearned for instant relief in any way, shape, or form it might be found.

"At this point in time, it was nearly impossible for me to even hold a clear thought! There was so much in life that I wanted to accomplish, yet my days were spent consulting doctors and lying on the couch wondering if I would ever get my life back. Looking back on the whole scenario, I can see clearly that there were no doctors available to me who could treat the whole me. Until my friend recommended homeopathy and Judyth.

"I am happy to report that I eventually did get my life back. It has been a gradual and sometimes agonizing process, but I would not trade the journey for anything. Today I work full time (what a blessing!), the allergies are abating slowly but surely, and my dependence on the high doses of medication has been reduced to the lowest possible doses. There may come a day when I do not need the medications at all. I have not had a seizure in ten years and the hormones I take, after years of adjustment and fine tuning, work beautifully.

"My life is working very well now and the most important aspect about all of this is that I FEEL GOOD. My body feels 'right.' It took a very long time before I could say that. Today I can support myself expressing the talent I love, I have wonderful friends and a delightful social life, and I have worked through a variety of childhood issues that had held me back. In the true spirit of treating the whole patient, my story, as I tell it now, shows me that homeopathy, in my case, has truly treated the whole me on all levels."

Laurie is a changed woman since I first met her in 1991. I would attribute her transformation, first, to her determination to heal no matter what, second, to homeopathy, which has helped her a great deal. She received *Staphysagria* (stavesacre), *Alumina* (aluminum), and *Natrum muriaticum* (sodium chloride) with considerable benefit until almost a year ago, when I changed her prescription to *Natrum phosphoricum* (sodium phosphate), which has helped her heal even more profoundly. Laurie has also received help from various forms of therapy.

When I first saw her, she had been on medication for seizures since age twelve. The convulsions terrified her, due to the violent jerking of her whole body. Gas and bloating were a major concern and, less so, recurrent sinus infections, bruising, and hemorrhoids. An ovarian cyst had prompted a total hysterectomy at the age of thirty-three, after which she had been placed on hormones and gained twenty pounds. Laurie had spent years trying to overcome a lifelong depression, history of drug and alcohol abuse, sexual abuse, fear of abandonment, and repeated feelings of rejection in intimate relationships. The beginning of Laurie's recovery, her recall of being abused, and her hysterectomy all occurred within a short period of time, leaving her confused and blind-sided.

Laurie has overcome most of her difficult past, as well as her physical, mental, and emotional problems. Most recently, she has needed *Natrum phosphoricum* due to her strong desire for support and affection, combined with her pattern of withdrawing into isolation when she feels rejected in a relationship. She now feels much better about herself, has less of a need to please people, and is no longer devastated if she doesn't receive the nurturing and support she seeks. Laurie is the first to admit that she still has a ways to go, but now that she's come as far as she has, she relishes the journey.

Karen's Story

"I am now perimenopausal. For a number of months, a year or two ago, I was having eight to nine days of period, then seven to ten days with no period, then back to eight to nine days of bleeding again. Some of it was spotting, some was like the flow of a regular period. I felt exhausted all the time. Whenever I saw Judyth for a visit (I tended to wait until my scheduled visits even though I knew I could call earlier), I was given a homeopathic medicine and, within a few weeks, I was back on a normal schedule with my periods.

"I choose not to have a medical doctor and have not been to one for many, many years. I am blessed with good health and I like to follow a more natural way of treating any problems that may arise. Homeopathy has been a wonderful way for me to go through menopause without having to deal with taking hormones or other medications. My hormone therapy is happening homeopathically! I believe, as I get older

(I am fifty-three now), that I will find a general practitioner, but homeopathy is what I prefer and I will continue to use it as a way of maintaining my well-being in harmony with the body, mind, and spirit."

Karen has had her share of gynecological problems, including extreme PMS, genital herpes, a miscarriage, irregular periods, and bleeding in between her periods, and, finally, she is approaching menopause. Though *Sepia* (cuttlefish ink) was extremely helpful to her for almost eight years, I changed her medicine to *Chocolate* a year ago.

Not only does Karen crave chocolate to the extreme, but it acts as a mood-altering substance for her (in her case, a downer). It was not unusual for Karen to eat most of a three-quarter pound bag of Hershey's kisses at one sitting. In fact, she calls herself a recovering chocolate addict! She did not feel that she received adequate nurturing by her mother and has suffered from loneliness, isolation, and a feeling that no one was there for her. Though Karen still continues to have her ups and downs, she is doing much better in all ways, thanks to homeopathy.

Description
Menopause is considered the time, usually around age fifty to fifty-two, but often earlier or later (anywhere between forty-five to fifty-five is common), when you have not had a period for one year. A number of hormonal symptoms may begin earlier, during perimenopause, even though you are still having periods.

Symptoms
In my experience, just about any symptom you've ever had can get worse, usually temporarily, during perimenopause, even symptoms that apparently have nothing to do with hormones. So, even if your doctor tells you, for example, that your itchy toe has absolutely nothing to do with your menopause, I wouldn't necessarily believe it. It is estimated that three-quarters of all menopausal women experience hot flashes and sweating to some extent. Whether or not or to what degree you go through other symptoms is up for grabs and depends on your mother's menopausal experience (by the time I asked my mom, she couldn't even remember when it occurred, much less the details); your habits, predispositions, and overall health; and perhaps your luck and your karma!

The most typical physical symptoms of the menopausal years are hot flashes or flushes; vaginal dryness, irritation, and fragility; headaches; fatigue; diminished sexual energy, headaches; odd sensations on the skin or anywhere else in the body (such as feeling you'll jump out of your skin); irregular periods; excessively heavy or scanty uterine bleeding; dry skin; insomnia; heart palpitations; painful sex; urinary incontinence; vaginal infections; skin problems; and a variety of digestive and musculoskeletal complaints, the most prominent of which is osteoporosis. That's quite a list, isn't it? It makes you understand why menopause is such a major concern for so many women! And why it is so important to go into it well-informed and in a positive frame of mind. Add to this the potential mental and emotional symptoms, such as irritability, depression, nervousness, mood swings, memory problems, confusion, and all that goes along with the change in roles, our bodies, our self-images, and the fact that we can no longer bear children.

Complications
The major "complications" are osteoporosis and heart disease, although there are a number of conditions, such as breast cancer, to which women are increasingly predisposed with age.

Conventional Treatment
The standard conventional treatment is estrogen replacement and, if you still have a uterus, progesterone replacement for at least part of the month to avoid the increased risk of uterine cancer caused by estrogen replacement. If you have a history of breast or any other estrogen-mediated cancer, estrogen replacement is definitely contraindicated and progestins appear to be as well. Consider yourself lucky if you do make it to menopause and beyond with your uterus intact because about half of women in the United States no longer have their uteruses by age sixty-five (although, in my experience, if you are a homeopathic patient and/or educated about your alternatives, your chances are immensely higher of avoiding a hysterectomy).

What to Expect from Homeopathic Treatment
Homeopathy is an excellent approach to menopause, regardless of what other therapies you use (although most homeopaths recommend against using acupuncture at the same time). It will very likely eliminate or minimize your hot flashes and other physical symptoms. Your libido may or may not be significantly improved with homeopathy alone, but, if it is not, you have the option of adding other conventional and/or alternative supplemental

therapies. I do not rely on homeopathy alone to prevent osteoporosis and heart disease and always recommend an integrated program of homeopathy, diet, and nutritional and often botanical supplements, as well an overall exercise and lifestyle program. I consider homeopathy to be a mainstay in an overall approach to well-being, during and after menopause.

Why You Need to Be Proactive Before Menopause

Do whatever reading, investigation, and laboratory tests that are appropriate to find out where you are on the menopausal spectrum. I do not recommend a wait-and-see approach to menopause for the following reasons:

• Some menopausal symptoms such as hot flashes, sleep problems, and mood changes can occur months or years before your flow actually stops and you will want to be as prepared as possible to make the best choices.

• A significant amount of bone loss, up to 10 percent, can occur in the first year after your period stops, then it continues steadily at a lower rate, say 2 to 3 percent a year. You want to develop a strategy to protect yourself *before* your bone loss begins.

• Hot flashes and vaginal dryness, not to mention all of the other symptoms women frequently experience during menopause, can be irritating and disturb your quality of life. You will surely want to increase your odds of sailing through, or at least effectively managing, these symptoms before or as soon as they occur.

• If you had a history of breast cancer, for example, and did not know to avoid estrogen replacement, you might end up with a recurrence.

• Menopause can be a tough time emotionally and can take a toll on career, relationships, and self-image. Homeopathy and other therapies, both alternative and conventional, can help you to go through the process with more ease and grace.

• You can choose to reframe menopause as a graceful period of transition and freedom rather than as a miserable time of your life.

• You have lots of choices and need to educate yourself and assess what is best for you. Women have more control over what happens to them at menopause than ever before, and it doesn't necessarily take a long time to become relatively expert about what you need.

Whether or Not to Take Hormones

A growing number of women in this country seem to be questioning whether synthetic hormone replacement is for them, which I applaud. If your doctor simply assumes that you will take hormones or that, now that you no longer wish to have a child, you no longer need your uterus, I strongly urge you to do your own research to find out what's right for you, talk to other women facing the same questions and decision, and possibly, find a new doctor.

What to Ask Yourself in Deciding Whether Hormone Replacement Is for You:

- At what age did I reach menopause? (Menopause prior to age forty is more of a compelling reason to take synthetic hormones.)
- What is my family history of osteoporosis?
- What is my family history of heart disease?
- Do I have a strong family history of Alzheimer's disease?
- Do I smoke? (This increases your risk of osteoporosis.)
- Do I drink more than a couple of glasses of alcohol a week? (This increases your risk of osteoporosis.)
- What is my body type? If you tend to be thin and small-boned and have dry skin, nervousness, insomnia, and gas, you are more disposed to osteoporosis. Ayurvedic medicine would classify you as having a Vata constitution. The recommendation is to drink lots of liquids, preferably warm or hot; include olive and/or canola oil in your diet; rub your body with sesame oil on a regular basis, avoid or minimize foods that give you gas, such as the cabbage family and beans; choose cooked over raw vegetables, avoid overstimulation; and relax.
- Do I have a history of fractures, bone weakness or surgery, bone loss in the gums, or any other indication of bone problems?
- Am I willing to eat a low-fat diet rich in whole grains, fiber, fresh and preferably organic fruits and vegetables, adequate protein, soy, and flax, and to minimize sugar, caffeine, alcohol, and pesticides?
- Am I willing to do aerobic and weight-bearing exercise for at least twenty minutes a minimum of three times a week?
- Have I taken any drugs associated with an increased risk of osteoporosis for an extended period of time (these include high doses of thyroid medication, steroids, and some diuretics)?
- Am I a positive, motivated person who is likely to lead a healthful lifestyle for the rest of my life?
- How long do I want to and am I likely to live?
- How active am I likely to be and for how long?
- How willing am I to accept aging?
- If I opt *not* to take hormone replacement, do I have the will, resources, and support to undertake a well-considered and balanced natural menopausal program?

If You Do Opt for Hormones, What Kind?

Contrary to your mother's options, or even those available to women five years ago, even if you do choose the hormone route in addition to homeopathy, there are a number of possibilities. If this is your path, I urge you to find a practitioner who thinks outside of the Premarin-Provera box and who has lots of experience with individualized hormone replacement programs.

Since my expertise lies in homeopathy, I prefer to run by the options so that you can discuss them with the women's health-care practitioner of your choice.

- Estrogen patches
- Natural progesterone cream (made from wild yam)
- Oral micronized progesterone (OMP)
- Estriol in an oral form or as a vaginal cream
- A formula of Premarin, Provera, and Estriol (of which there are a number of combinations and permutations, such as tri-est and bi-est)
- DHEA
- Testosterone, orally or as a cream

For an in-depth discussion of the pros and cons of these various natural and synthetic hormones, refer to the highly informative *Women's Encyclopedia of Natural Medicine* by my naturopathic colleague Tori Hudson, N.D., or *Women's Bodies, Women's Minds* by Christine Northrup, M.D.

 Naturopathic Suggestions to Complement Homeopathic Care

- Eat a diet high in whole grains, fiber, fresh fruits and vegetables and with adequate protein.
- If heart disease, high triglycerides, or weight gain despite vigorous exercise is a problem, seriously consider the Zone Diet, or another diet that balances carbohydrates.
- Eat lots of soy products. (There is some controversy about how much soy to include if you have a history of breast cancer, so I will leave this up to you to research.)
- Eliminate caffeine and tobacco.
- Keep alcohol and sugar at a minimum.
- Take one tablespoon a day of ground flaxseeds or flaxseed oil.
- Eat salmon, mackerel, tuna, herring, halibut, and sardines and/or take fish oil capsules.
- Take a high-quality megamultivitamin and mineral containing 3 milligrams of boron.

- Take 1,200 milligrams of calcium citrate or the equivalent of calcium citrate malate (600 milligrams for the product that I use) and half of the amount of magnesium in the form of citrate or citrate malate.
- Add 400 to 800 IU of vitamin E.
- Take vitamin C, 1,000 milligrams or more a day.
- Soy isoflavones and ipriflavone (a synthetic derivative of isoflavones) appear to prevent bone loss.
- Do weight-bearing and aerobic exercise at least twenty minutes a day, three times a week.
- Many women use topical progesterone cream.
- Herbs that can be very helpful during menopause are black cohosh, chaste tree, and dong quai (I use them with my patients as part of a multivitamin/mineral product), as well as gingko (for memory problems).
- Take time to intentionally reevaluate your life so that you can make this new phase of your life healthful, productive, rewarding, full of love and fun, and enlightening.
- Get involved in a women's group of some kind to share your wisdom, experiences, and challenges with like-minded souls.

Menstrual Problems (Chronic)

Joy's Story

"When I first arrived in the Seattle area ten years ago, I had already experienced twenty-five years of debilitating period pains. From early adulthood, I would virtually collapse each month, destabilized from cramps that would force me to double over in excruciating pain and to vomit.

"It was a great relief when a good friend suggested that I try homeopathy, a painless process of sharing very intimate and seemingly disconnected information in the search for a cure that connects all the threads of one's life. This was surely preferable to a medical doctor poking and prodding to identify possible reasons for my pain.

"When I first met Judyth, I was quite amazed at the length of the initial consultation and by the questions she asked. Even more surprising was her saying at the end of the interview that she thought she had a way of helping me. As she described the medicine I needed as coming from the venom of a South American snake, my already fertile imagination was engaged, and I began to work internally with images connecting the divine feminine archetypes of the Snake Goddess and feminine wisdom and power. It made sense that such a vibration could address the many symptoms I had, all on the left side. The sensitivity of my nervous system, as well as my rich and rather dramatic emotional life, also seemed to fit the medicine she had selected.

"I took the medicine and my very next period was almost totally free of pain. It was an amazing turn of events and my life was significantly changed for the better. I have taken this medicine from time to time over the past ten years, with regular visits to Judyth as my schedule and travels from Europe allow. I can sense when I need another dose because everything gets intensified and, gradually, the harsh symptoms return. Once the medicine is renewed, things stabilize again and my cycles return to a place where I simply feel the pulse of the cramping without being overwhelmed by pain.

"I consider Judyth to be my primary health-care provider and am so grateful for the intervention of homeopathy. The standard medical model typically works on a gross level, but the subtle vibrational level is far more effective in producing long-lasting cures. Homeopathy seems to engage the spirit in a way that honors the whole being and that is true health care. Thank you."

It was truly a blessing for both of us that Joy discovered homeopathy. A blessing for me because Joy is one of the most powerful, centered, and clear women I have ever met, and she makes a tremendous impact on the world. A blessing for her because *Lachesis* (bushmaster snake) phenomenally improved her menstrual cramps and other symptoms.

The indications for *Lachesis* were incapacitating menstrual pain with vomiting, left ovarian pain, left-sided chest pain, oral herpes, and a dramatic, powerful nature. Women needing this medicine are intense and expressive and can suffer terribly if their avenues of expression, on any level, are blocked. Over the eight years that I have worked with Joy, she has needed nine doses of the *Lachesis*. Like a fine wine, she improves with age.

Description

You may experience a variety of menstrual problems. The two main ones are abnormal periods and painful periods (dysmenorrhea). Abnormal menstrual bleeding (which, aside from bleeding related to cancer or the absence of periods, is often lumped in the category of dysfunctional uterine bleeding, or DUB) includes:

- bleeding that occurs according to your normal cycle but is excessively heavy (menorrhagia)
- bleeding that is normal in quantity but occurs between your periods (metrorrhagia) and may last for days or weeks at a time
- irregular periods

- cycles that are unusually long or short
- extremely light periods (hypomenorrhea)
- an absence of menstrual periods (amenorrhea)

Some degree of cramping or pain with your periods is normal, but excessive, or even debilitating pain, is not. Pain associated with the menses may be confined to the pelvic area and abdomen or may involve the lower back or legs. If your pain is severe, you may be confined to bed for a day or so each month. A number of other symptoms, including fatigue, constipation or diarrhea, headache, nausea with or without vomiting, chills, and increased urinary frequency, may accompany menstrual pain.

Symptoms

The range of variation in menstruation can be vast. If your periods are excessively heavy, it is common to have clotting and pain. If your periods are irregular, you may or may not be ovulating and I recommend that you learn to track your cycle by means of your temperature and cervical mucus in order to find out if and when you do ovulate. You may experience spotting or, if your periods are unusually heavy due to a number of possible reasons, you may find yourself bleeding continuously for weeks at a time. Difficulty in becoming pregnant can also be a result of abnormal periods.

Complications

Anemia, mild to severe, can occur if your bleeding is excessive and prolonged. In extreme cases, unmonitored blood loss over a long period of time can cause an iron loss so significant that you could even die. Uterine cancer needs to be ruled out if bleeding persists. The other common complication of menstrual abnormalities is infertility.

Conventional Treatment

Orthodox treatment for abnormal menstrual bleeding usually falls into four categories:

- hormones
- surgery, varying from a D & C (dilation and curettage), in which the uterine lining is scraped, to endometrial ablation (a partial or total hysterectomy)
- drugs to control associated symptoms such as menstrual pain
- nutritional supplementation such as iron, to reverse anemia

What to Expect from Homeopathic Treatment

I have found homeopathy to be an excellent treatment for all aspects of menstrual problems.

- Excessively heavy periods: flow should become normal.
- Irregular periods: cycles will come closer to every twenty-eight days, according to what is normal for *you.*
- Scanty periods will become heavier.
- Periods that are primarily brown in color will become brighter red.
- Length of periods will generally become three to seven days rather than very short or long.
- Clotting will diminish.
- Menstrual pain will disappear or improve significantly.
- Women who have no periods may begin to have them.

In general, homeopathy is highly effective for menstrual problems and moderately effective for initiating periods when there have been none, depending on the cause of the amenorrhea.

Naturopathic Suggestions to Complement Homeopathic Care

For all kinds of menstrual problems:

- Eat more cold-water fish such as salmon, sardines, tuna, herring, and halibut and less of animal products like red meat and dairy products.
- If you eat poultry, make sure it's free of hormones and antibiotics.
- Daily calcium supplementation of 1,000 milligrams often decreases or relieves cramps.
- Take vitamin E, 400 to 800 IU a day.
- Take evening primrose, black currant, borage, or fish oils.
- Use natural progesterone cream.
- Do regular aerobic exercise.
- Practice yoga postures specifically geared to balancing uterine function.

For menstrual cramps:

- Follow all of the previous recommendations.
- Niacin (vitamin B_3) can be very helpful in relieving menstrual pain if you take 100 milligrams twice a day on an ongoing basis and 100 milligrams every few hours when you actually have the acute pain (you will probably notice a temporary niacin flush).
- Crampbark is an herb that is well-known to help with menstrual pain and valerian root can help relax you and decrease spasms of the uterus.

- Take a sitz bath. Fill the tub with hot water up to two inches below your navel. Sit with your knees bent. Stay in the tub for five minutes. Then squat in a tub of cold water for one minute. Repeat the cycle two to three times.
- Avoid using tampons if they make your periods more painful.

Miscarriages *(Recurrent)*

Ruth's Story

"At the time I first sought the help of Dr. Reichenberg-Ullman, I was forty-one years old and in good health except for the fact that I was unable to sustain a pregnancy beyond four to eight weeks. Although I had no trouble conceiving naturally, I had suffered four first-trimester miscarriages over the course of the previous four years. I felt fine during all of my pregnancies and followed a healthful lifestyle with no smoking, drinking, or fast foods; lots of vegetables; moderate exercise; and a happy home and work life. This made my situation even harder for me to understand.

"Under the care of my ob-gyn and a geneticist, numerous tests were performed on both me and my husband, as well as on the 'products of conception.' Afterward, we were told only that no explanation could be found. This, needless to say, compounded my level of frustration. I am the type of person who researches everything to the nth degree, and even with my additional investigation, I came up with no answers.

"At this point I felt ready to seek a medical alternative, as long as it was not too radical. Through a friend I heard of homeopathy and Dr. Reichenberg-Ullman and decided to explore it further. Though I lived across the country from Washington State, I was assured that as long as I was under medical care locally, she could treat me long-distance.

"At the very same time, I learned of a fertility specialist who had recently joined my doctor's clinic and was reported to have a record of excellent results. After reviewing my case, the specialist recommended a laparoscopy and hysteroscopy to investigate further. I agreed. Upon my discussing the decision to have surgical procedures with Dr. Reichenberg-Ullman, she outlined a protocol of homeopathic medicines and nutritional supplements to facilitate a speedy recuperation with minimal scar tissue afterward. Then I was to take a constitutional homeopathic medicine that she believed fit me well.

"The surgery revealed scar tissue in my uterus (previously undetected and of unknown source), which they removed. My recuperation was quick and painless. I then took the homeopathic medicine, which was *Arsenicum album*. The changes weren't dramatic, except for a more positive outcome in my recurrent dreams, but then again, I didn't really have any complaints except for the miscarriages.

"Within a few months I was pregnant again. This time, however, I continued to full term (actually nine days beyond!), unlike all of my other pregnancies, with absolutely no problems. Despite a very hot summer, I experienced no swelling, minimal weight gain, and a relatively quick vaginal delivery, which resulted in a beautiful, healthy baby boy."

I gave Ruth *Arsenicum album* (arsenic) based primarily on her caution and orderliness. Her parents had been overprotective and didn't allow her to sleep over at friends' houses. Ruth really didn't need to take many risks in her life, so it didn't get much in the way of her happiness. A logical, methodical, and organized woman, Ruth's work, marriage, family, and life in general were in order and worked quite well for her. The only thing she wanted help with was maintaining a pregnancy until its happy conclusion.

There is no way of knowing exactly how much the surgery helped versus the homeopathy. What is important is that five and a half months after beginning homeopathy, Ruth conceived and successfully had a beautiful baby boy right on schedule. I also prescribed *Arsenicum album* for her morning sickness.

My Own Story

"I, unfortunately, experienced five miscarriages in five years. None of the health professionals I consulted, whether conventional or alternative, could ever figure out the cause and I was not able to carry a pregnancy beyond sixteen weeks. However, homeopathy helped me with my third miscarriage and was a lifesaver during my fifth.

"My pain was not so severe the third time and I actually went through the cramping and passed the fetus while at the home of some close friends. I felt quite weak afterward and felt my energy return after a dose of *China* (Peruvian bark), an excellent homeopathic medicine for depletion following loss of blood or other bodily fluids.

"My fifth and final miscarriage was the worst. I cannot even describe the pain except to say it must be like having gone through labor but not ending up with your baby. Waves of the most stabbing uterine pain came every few minutes, causing me to scream out, which only relieved the pain for a split second. Oral Demoral didn't touch it. I was in so much agony that at one point, an image went through my mind of plunging a knife into my uterus to end the pain. Not that I would have done it, but that was my desperation with such unrelenting pain. That agony led me to a take *Aurum metallicum* (gold) which can alleviate terrible, deep pains that cause someone to want to die. Within five minutes of taking the *Aurum,* the pain began to diminish and was much more bearable until I passed the fetus an hour or so later."

Description

Miscarriage, also known as spontaneous abortion, is defined as the loss of a pregnancy before the twentieth week. Up to 30 percent of women have some cramping or bleeding during this stage of their pregnancy, with 10 to 15 percent suffering a miscarriage. Though it is estimated that in 60 percent of miscarriages, the fetus is absent or deformed in some way, the experience, nevertheless, can be very traumatic, particular when it is recurrent.

Symptoms

Symptoms vary considerably, depending to a large extent on how far along you are when it occurs, and can range from mild cramping and bleeding to severe and incapacitating laborlike pains.

Complications

The worst-case scenario is a septic abortion in which the contents of the uterus develop an infection, either before or after the miscarriage, which can result in shock or death.

Conventional Treatment

In most cases, you cannot stop a miscarriage from occurring; however, bed rest is recommended and will, at times, allow the pregnancy to continue to full term. In the case of an incompetent cervix, cerclage is a surgical procedure that holds the cervix in place to allow the pregnancy to continue. Once a miscarriage occurs, pain pills and a D & C (dilation and curettage) are the conventional mode of treatment. In cases of late-stage miscarriage, the woman must go on to deliver the dead fetus.

What to Expect from Homeopathic Treatment

If you tend toward recurrent miscarriages, homeopathy can help bring you into balance so that you can potentially complete healthy pregnancies, as in Ruth's case.

Naturopathic Suggestions to Complement Homeopathic Care

• Eat a nutritious diet, take a high-quality prenatal vitamin and mineral supplement, exercise, and take care of yourself to ensure as healthy a pregnancy as possible.

- Avoid foods made from unpasteurized milk, soft cheeses such as Brie, and undercooked meat, poultry, and seafood, which can spread listerium bacteria that often cause miscarriages.
- If you do begin to miscarry, take it easy or go to bed and let nature take its course.
- If you are in extreme pain, call your doctor or homeopath immediately for appropriate help.
- Express your emotions openly and honestly so that healing can occur.
- Ask your doctor if there is any clear cause for the miscarriage, to ease your mind about it happening again in the future.
- Treat a miscarriage as the death in the family that it is and let yourself be comforted.
- Realize that friends and family may not know how approach you or what to say, and don't take it personally.
- Get help in the form of counseling or a support group if you need it.

Mood Swings

Debbie's Story

"I can hardly believe where I was and where I am today. After suffering so many years from severe mood swings and debilitating migraines, I had nearly given up hope. I came to Dr. Reichenberg-Ullman as a last resort. I don't honestly think I expected anything near the dramatic results I experienced. I feel really free for the first time. I don't know how I lasted as long as I did. I guess we can get used to the worst if it creeps up slowly enough. I tell my story to anyone who indicates the slightest interest!"

Debbie had a total hysterectomy eleven months before I first saw her. She had experienced heavy clotting due to uterine fibroids. Earlier in her life, she been treated with hormones due to heavy and erratic menstrual bleeding, "like a floodgate." Her sexual energy now was "below zero." She was on Premarin since the hysterectomy.

Her mood swings were extreme, ranging from a hyper phase lasting several days at time during which she accomplished superhuman tasks. Then she would hit the wall, feel normal for a week, then the cycle would begin again. During her more infrequent down phases, Debbie wanted to be left alone, felt devoid of energy, and was in bed by 7 P.M. She was enveloped in hopelessness, helplessness, and a sense of foreboding.

Debbie suffered from incapacitating migraines. There was an extensive history of cancer in her family, which led her to fear that she, too, would develop a malignancy.

She had recently consulted a dermatologist and had had a dark mole removed. Though it was benign, she had read all the literature on malignant melanoma.

Carcinosin (nosode) had a profound effect on Debbie. Her migraines disappeared, as did all of her physical symptoms, including blisters on the sclera of her eyes and fibrocystic breasts (which had bothered her for the previous five years), and her moods stabilized. Debbie has only recently returned for treatment after needing no homeopathic care for six years.

Description

Mood swings are erratic, often unpredictable shifts in emotions. There are a number of causes of mood swings; one of the most common in women is hormonal ups and downs.

Symptoms

Symptoms run the gamut of the emotional spectrum, ranging from grief to joy, anger to ecstasy, and calmness to anguish, often changing dramatically within hours or even minutes.

Your partner or loved ones may only half-jokingly say they can't predict which one of you they are likely to find. Mood swings, when severe, can get in the way of relationships, work, and life in general.

Complications

The most serious complication is harm to oneself or others, even homicide or suicide.

Conventional Treatment

Drug therapy depends on the diagnosis and ranges from anti-anxiety medications and antidepressants to medications such as lithium carbonate for bipolar disorder.

What to Expect from Homeopathic Treatment

Homeopathy can be highly effective for mild to moderate mood disorders and effective in some cases of bipolar disorder (see *Prozac-Free* for cases of bipolar disorder and other mood disorders successfully treated with homeopathy).

Naturopathic Suggestions to Complement Homeopathic Care

- Eat a high-quality, balanced diet high in whole grains, fruits, vegetables, and fiber.
- If your mood swings are at all related to hypoglycemia, be sure you eat plenty of protein; limit concentrated sources of simple carbohydrates such as juice, dried fruits, and sweets; and don't go too long without eating.
- Some women find St. John's wort, 300 milligrams three times a day, helpful for depression, or SAMe for depression with or without joint pain.
- For anxiety, herbs such as passionflower, valerian, skullcap, hops, and chamomile can be quite helpful.
- Put as much routine in your life as possible, to make things predictable and constant.
- Take one day at a time and put your energy into what is most important in your life and what you really can change, and let the rest go.
- Spend time with people who are calm and can help you feel more balanced.
- Some excellent short-term psychotherapy techniques, such as rapid eye movement, thought field therapy, NLP (neurolinguistic programming), and Ericksonian hypnosis, can be great aids to stabilizing moods.
- Every time you feel your mood going out of control, imagine or visualize tendrils going down from your navel to the center of the earth. Continue to breathe in and out until you feel more grounded.
- Regular aerobic exercise, especially in fresh air, is a good calming device.
- Yoga, meditation, contemplation, and prayer are excellent tools for centering.

Morning Sickness (Severe or Persistent)

Anna's Story

"I was so looking forward to my third and final pregnancy. Having gone through it twice before, I thought this one would be a breeze. A piece of cake. I was definitely wrong! Almost immediately the morning sickness set in. I had suffered morning sickness for the initial ten weeks of my first pregnancy and virtually none with my second child. So, as my pregnancy progressed beyond fourteen weeks and I was still four pounds lighter than when I began, I knew I had to do something fast! Driving was impossible unless I carried a bag into which I could vomit. Pop Tarts and Ramen Noodles were my survival diet.

"Conventional medicine does not offer a completely safe option for morning sickness. My obstetrician prescribed Hydroxyzine to help with the nausea, but it offered only temporary relief with no guarantee that it would not harm my baby. I saw Judyth during my fourteenth week of pregnancy. After an hour-long interview, she prescribed *Colchicum*. Within the next two weeks, my morning sickness diminished and I gained six pounds.

"Six weeks later, I went back to see her. Though physically much better, I felt like I was riding an emotional roller coaster with no brakes. Judyth gave me another dose of the same medicine. Within forty-eight hours, I felt like my normal self.

"During my eighth month of pregnancy, I once more experienced morning sickness, coupled with muscle pain in my shoulder, loose bowel movements, and sleeplessness. Again she repeated the *Colchium* and, as before, I felt immediate relief.

"I can't explain why *Colchium* can cure morning sickness, pregnancy blues, muscle pain, loose bowel movements, and sleeplessness. Nor why the medicines Judyth gave me for mastitis and all three of my children for a variety of physical and behavioral problems have worked so consistently and beautifully. I can only say, 'IT WORKS!'"

Anna is one of the most engaging and delightful women I have ever met—down-home, friendly, and vivacious. And her children, whom I also treat, are equally lively, especially since her daughter has received the right homeopathic medicine. Anna came to see me for the first time nearly a year ago when she was thirteen and a half weeks pregnant. She was beset with a horrible gagging sensation as soon as she smelled, looked at, or even thought about food. Her stomach felt achy and full of gas bubbles. The gagging occurred about six times a day and vomiting two to three times daily. Anna had experienced similar symptoms while pregnant with her son but not as severe or long-lasting. She also had what she described as a "weird thing with her toes," which turned out to be Raynaud's syndrome (incredible coldness and a purplish discoloration). She even had to wear socks at night to get to sleep.

Colchicum (meadow saffron) made the rest of Anna's pregnancy a joy. She needed a total of four doses over the course of five months until she delivered an adorable baby and then again shortly after the birth for thrush and continued uterine bleeding. The *Colchicum* has worked like a charm every time. It is interesting to note that *Colchicum* and its synthetic derivative, colchine, are excellent medicines for gout, of which purplish toes can be a symptom.

Description
Morning sickness is nausea, with or without vomiting, that can put a damper on the first few months, or even the entire duration of your pregnancy.

Symptoms

Mild to incapacitating nausea with aversion to the sight, smell, and sometimes the mere idea of food is common. A variety of factors can aggravate the nausea, including motion, eating, drinking, and emotional upset.

Complications

Other than the discomfort, inconvenience, and disappointment, the biggest complication of prolonged morning sickness is malnutrition and inability to gain sufficient weight. If extreme and long-lasting, it can sometimes result in low birth weight and other problems for the newborn. Hyperemesis gravidarum—severe and unremitting vomiting during pregnancy, which may be associated with liver disease—can cause dehydration and necessitate hospitalization and intravenous fluids.

Conventional Treatment

Antinausea medications are prescribed by conventional physicians and, in extreme cases, intravenous fluids are given.

What to Expect from Homeopathic Treatment

I don't believe I've ever seen a case of morning sickness that didn't respond favorably to homeopathy within seven to ten days.

Naturopathic Suggestions to Complement Homeopathic Care

• Try out different combinations of food to see if any of them agrees with you.
• Eat small amounts of food often.
• Have a snack by your bed to munch on before you get out of bed in the morning.
• Saltine crackers can relieve the nausea.
• You are likely to prefer bland foods such as broth, rice, and pasta.
• Tea and toast are usually well-tolerated.
• Ginger root tea can often relieve the nausea of morning sickness. Boil a one-quarter-inch slice of fresh ginger root in a cup of water for fifteen minutes. Strain and drink.
• Take your prenatal vitamins with meals. You may need to cut down the dosage during morning sickness, but try to get at least some of them down.
• Stimulating Stomach 36, an acupressure point in the soft area below the knee and to the outside of the leg where the tibia and fibula bones meet, is

often helpful for nausea. Use firm rotary pressure on the spot for a few seconds and repeat as often as necessary.

Osteoporosis

Darlene's Story

"I am a seventy-one-year-old woman and have suffered from severe depression and osteoporosis and osteoarthritis for forty-five years. I have had several broken bones, four pelvic fractures, seven spinal fractures, and five fractures of the tibia and fibula.

"Having been under the care of Dr. Reichenberg-Ullman for four years, I have found that the homeopathic treatment has greatly helped me. My mobility is much better and the pain is drastically reduced."

I've known Darlene, a retired accountant in Florida, for four years, since she was sixty-seven. The one thing that stands out most in my mind about her is that she is a lady in the finest sense of the word. But Darlene has really been through it: colon cancer, a husband who left her for another woman, hypertension, and osteoporosis, as well as a deep depression.

It has been a challenge to find a medicine that would make a profound difference for Darlene. The one that has been most helpful and has produced a definite decrease in her pain and facilitated her getting around more easily is *Calcarea fluorica* (calcium fluoride). It is a great remedy for fractures and for a feeling of having lost one's source of security and support. Some people tend to fear that their financial foundation will be eroded and this is what happens to their body as well.

Darlene's case is still very much in progress and it remains to be seen just how much homeopathy can help her osteoporosis. All along she has been taking other conventional medications and nutritional supplements for her bones without significant improvement, and with a variety of side effects, so the fact that she has felt so much better after the *Calcarea fluorica* is encouraging.

Description

Osteoporosis is a progressive loss of mass in the bone tissue, resulting in weakness of the skeleton. This condition affects 25 million people and causes 1.5 million fractures each year, resulting in osteoporosis-related fractures in half of all women over the age of sixty-five.[4] It is particularly common, though not limited to women after menopause, and may be aggravated by certain substances such as steroids, alcohol, tobacco, barbiturates, and high doses of thyroid medication.

Symptoms

You may have no symptoms at all, or you may experience aching in your bones, especially your back. Fractures, as a result of osteoporosis, most often affect the spine, hip, and forearm. If you develop a fracture of your mid- or lower vertebrae, you may notice a tenderness in that area. In severe cases of osteoporosis, the pain can be debilitating.

Complications

The most significant result of osteoporosis are fractures, which often, especially in the case of hip fractures, require hospitalization and recovery in a nursing home. Women's overall mobility, health, well-being, and quality of life often begin to deteriorate at this point, sometimes permanently.

Conventional Treatment

Orthodox medicine usually recommends estrogen/progestin supplementation and Fossamax, which inhibits resorption of the bone. The newest medication is raloxifene, a type of selective estrogen receptor modulator, which is said to increase bone density without stimulating growth of the endometrial uterine tissue like Tamoxifen.

What Can You Expect from Homeopathic Treatment?

Given the serious repercussions of osteoporosis and the lack of conclusive research on the treatment of osteoporosis with homeopathy alone, I recommend a program including homeopathy, diet, nutritional supplementation, exercise, and, if appropriate for you, hormone-replacement therapy. With such a combined regimen, your chances are good, unless you are at high risk, to avoid significant bone loss.

The following characteristics put you at a greater risk for osteoporosis.

After menopause:
- Short stature, fair skin, thin and wiry build, small-boned.
- Early menopause (either natural or surgery- or drug-induced).
- No full-term pregnancies.
- Family history of osteoporosis.

- History of missed periods or infrequent periods or lack of ovulation.
- Tendency toward fractures or bone loss.
- High intake of animal proteins, caffeine, and salt.
- Low calcium and high phosphorus (meat and carbonated drinks) intake.
- Smoking
- Moderate or excessive alcohol intake.
- Sedentary lifestyle.
- Prolonged use of steroids, seizure medications, aluminum-containing antacids, antitubercular medicines, heparin, and tetracycline.
- Removal of intestines or both lobes of thyroid.

Naturopathic Suggestions to Complement Homeopathic Care

- Eat a diet high in whole grains, fresh fruits and vegetables, adequate protein (limit the animal sources), and fiber.
- Include calcium-rich seaweed in your diet.
- Drink at least six glasses of water a day.
- What is your body type? If you tend to be thin and small-boned and have dry skin, nervousness, insomnia, and gas, you are more disposed to osteoporosis. Ayurvedic medicine would classify you as having a Vata constitution. The recommendation is to drink lots of liquids, preferably warm or hot; include olive and/or canola oil in your diet; rub your body with sesame oil on a regular basis; avoid or minimize foods that give you gas, such as the cabbage family and beans; choose cooked over raw vegetables.
- Minimize carbonated drinks (high in phosphorus), sugar, and salt.
- Avoid caffeine and tobacco.
- Avoid or minimize alcohol.
- Stay at the optimal weight for you. Being too thin predisposes you to osteoporosis more than being too heavy.
- Take a daily, high-quality megamultivitamin and mineral supplement, including vitamin D, 800 IU; magnesium citrate malate, 300 milligrams; vitamin K, 250–500 micrograms; and boron, 3 milligrams.
- Take 1,200 milligrams a day of calcium citrate or 600 milligrams a day of calcium citrate malate or another highly absorbable calcium.
- Make soy isoflavones and ipriflavone a part of your diet.
- Do weight-bearing exercise, particularly weight lifting, for at least twenty minutes, three times a week, in addition to cardiovascular exercise.

Ovarian Cysts and Polycystic Ovaries

Ginny's Story

At forty-five, Ginny, a patient of my husband, Bob, was found to have a left ovarian cyst on a routine pelvic exam, and it was confirmed by ultrasound to be quite large (eight centimeters). During the examination, prior to the ultrasound, her gynecologist had scared her to death by saying it might be ovarian cancer. She had missed a period two months before, and her last period was quite heavy. Ginny complained of aching pain in her abdomen from mid-cycle to the middle of her period.

At the same time, Ginny had to care for her disabled sister, who had been recently cut off by their mother, which caused her to feel devastated and broken-hearted. She described it as a bombardment of "negative feminine energy" from her family. Ginny also had an incident with a coworker in which she felt betrayed and a loss of trust.

Ginny had always had a strong fear of snakes since her brother had startled her with one when she was a child. Now she couldn't even think of a snake without feeling frightened. The left-sided cyst, along with her feeling of betrayal and fear of snakes, led to the prescription of *Lachesis* (bushmaster snake). One month later, Ginny reported feeling "absolutely fantastic." The first day after taking the medicine she said she actually felt like a snake. Within the next six weeks, the left ovarian cyst had shrunk to less than one centimeter; however, two small, new cysts had been discovered on the right ovary, each one centimeter in diameter. Ginny experienced her first normal, cramp-free, seven-day period in a long time. Her fear of snakes diminished. Within two and a half months after taking the *Lachesis,* her gynecologist informed her that all of the cysts were gone. Ginny was now able to resolve the issues with her sister and mother and was able to feel a new sense of inner peace. She needed one more repetition of *Lachesis* six months after the original prescription, when a few of her symptoms returned after she drank coffee.

Gail's Story

Gail, also a patient of my husband, Bob, had just been given *Phosphorus* for a variety of problems over a three-month period. Then, when she was seven weeks pregnant, her obstetrician found a mass in her abdomen measuring five inches in diameter. It was diagnosed on pelvic ultrasound as a midline corpus luteal cyst, and surgery was recommended in order to save the pregnancy. Gail was not thrilled with the idea of surgery and wanted to avoid it if at all possible.

Bob waited a month to see if the cyst would shrink from the *Phosphorus,* but it did not and her obstetrician urged her even more vehemently to have it removed because it endangered the pregnancy. Gail feared that the surgery posed an even greater risk and implored Bob to try another homeopathic medicine.

She described a pulling sensation on the right side that felt worse when she lay on it. Bob felt that the problem with lying on her right side, as well as a right-sided tonsillar swelling and a few other symptoms, were features of *Lycopodium* (club moss). Fortunately, his prescription worked. Within one week the cyst was half its former size and within two weeks it was gone.

Gail continued to have a healthy pregnancy, with the exception of catching one cold, with a right-sided sore throat and cough, also successfully treated with *Lycopodium*. Although corpus luteal cysts can resolve without treatment, the speed at which they diminished was surprising to Gail's obstetrician, who was glad that surgery could be avoided.

Description

Ovarian cysts are fluid-filled or solid cysts in the ovary, usually follicular or corpus luteal, and they usually resolve on their own in a month or two. Polycystic ovaries is a hormonal imbalance resulting in an excess of androgens and the failure of the ovaries to produce eggs.

Symptoms

Ovarian cysts are frequently asymptomatic but can also cause discomfort, tenderness, aching, heaviness, or severe pain. There may also be bleeding. The three main characteristics of polycystic ovaries are infertility, facial hair, and often excess weight.

Complications

The main complications of ovarian cysts are torsion (twisting), which can cause hemorrhage inside the abdomen; shock; peritonitis; and death. It is very important to differentiate between a benign ovarian mass and ovarian cancer, which generally necessitates removing and biopsying the ovary. The most disturbing complication associated with polycystic ovaries is infertility.

Conventional Treatment

The initial approach to ovarian cysts is often to wait and see what happens for a couple of months unless there is a suspicion of ovarian cancer or the cyst arises during pregnancy.

Birth control pills are the treatment of choice. Polycystic ovaries, if the symptoms are limited to hair growth, are also treated with birth control pills; however, more aggressive hormonal regimens are used if the woman wishes to become pregnant.

What to Expect from Homeopathic Treatment

Homeopathy can be helpful for ovarian cysts, generally within one to three months after taking the correct medicine. You should allow a minimum of six months to a year to see results with polycystic ovaries.

Naturopathic Suggestions to Complement Homeopathic Care

- Eat a diet high in whole grains, fresh fruits, vegetables, and fiber.
- Minimize or avoid red meat and dairy products.
- Drink at least six glasses of water a day.
- If you eat poultry, make sure it's free of hormones and antibiotics.
- Avoid caffeine.
- Avoid or minimize alcohol.
- Do not smoke.
- Take a daily, high-quality megamultivitamin and mineral supplement, including 300 milligrams magnesium citrate malate.
- Take 1,200 milligrams a day of calcium citrate or, preferably, 600 milligrams a day of calcium citrate malate.
- Lipotropic factors, particularly in combination with liver herbs such as dandelion root and milk thistle, can help the liver break down estrogen.
- Explore and clear any inner obstacles to releasing the cyst(s).

Pelvic Pain

Bri's Story

"When I began homeopathy in 1994, I had been suffering from a variety of problems, most of which were gynecological. The one that disturbed me the most was recurrent pelvic pain, to the point of being unable or unwilling to have sex. Because I had been treated in the past for venereal warts, I became paranoid about any vaginal discharge and was terrified to go to the gynecologist. I had suffered from abnormal Pap smears most of my adult life, even when I was barely sexually active.

"I also was bothered by skin problems, which seemed to coincide with hormonal changes but didn't ever clear up. I was rashy and red a lot of the time, and it seemed to take quite a while to heal from any outbreak. My skin was sallow. It was like perpetual PMS. My breasts were sore and I felt bloated and emotional most of the time. Then there were the despondency and lethargy. At times, I convinced myself that I was going to die.

"Homeopathy initially did two things for me. It gave me a feeling that I was doing something for myself that was not invasive, unlike the treatments I had endured at the gynecologist's for my warts. It also made me acknowledge myself as a person who is sensitive to substances such as coffee and drugs and who needs to refrain from using things that knock me off balance. I had consumed (or rather abused) caffeine for a number of years and still felt the effects. After I stopped drinking coffee and tea for good, it was still a long road to coming back into balance energy-wise. But I noticed, with the help of homeopathy from Judyth, that I was able to control my moods better and felt as if I had some will to live, even if I acknowledged that I was feeling down. I stopped getting so caught up in my negative feelings.

"Everything improved: my pelvic pain, vaginal discharge, PMS, energy, and mood. Of course, I fell back into drinking coffee a few times. Each time I felt worse and needed to call Judyth to have my medicine repeated. Whenever I increased my coffee consumption, I gradually watched many of my symptoms return with a vengeance.

"I believe that homeopathy is probably the only way for me to contend with conditions to which I seem particularly prone and with my behavior that makes them even more likely to occur. I think that the feeling of being a "fragile woman" is totally tied to my having a sensitive system that benefits from homeopathy's guiding balance. When I allow my fear to surface about having gynecological disease or distress, I am aware that it undercuts much of my power to function as a woman in this world."

I first met Bri four and a half years ago. At that time she was in her late twenties and her main problem was a history of abnormal Pap smears due to HPV. She suffered from vaginal and ovarian pain, a cottage-cheeselike vaginal discharge, and pain with sex, as well as fibrocystic breasts and a couple of wartlike eruptions on her labia. Mood swings, a high degree of sensitivity, self-doubt, and nervousness in social situations all got in the way of her expressing her full potential, both personally and artistically.

The medicine that helped Bri quite significantly was *Medorrhinum* (nosode). She finds it quite a challenge to stay away from coffee, but as long as the medicine is working, her vaginal discharge and discomfort are much better, her pelvic pain is considerably better, and she is much more at ease talking to people. Bri is in a loving relationship and is much happier with herself than before beginning homeopathy.

Description

Pain in the pelvic area, generally of gynecological or gastrointestinal origin, can be caused by a variety of problems, ranging from menstrual pain, ectopic pregnancy, miscarriage, ovarian cysts, uterine fibroids, endometriosis, pelvic inflammatory disease (inflammation and/or abscess of the fallopian tubes, better known as PID), HIV infection, or cancer to appendicitis, gallbladder problems, intestinal obstruction, and many others. Pelvic inflammatory disease can result from sexually transmitted diseases, such as gonorrhea or chlamydia, or from infections caused by IUDs or cervical sponges, or can follow abortions.

Symptoms

Pelvic pain can be mild or severe. When I was in medical school, I was taught that the main finding to confirm pelvic inflammatory disease was "the chandelier sign," in which the woman suffers such excruciating pain on physical examination that she screams and reaches for the ceiling. This gives some idea of how severe the pain can be.

Complications

The most severe complication of pelvic inflammatory disease is shock, peritonitis, and death. Other complications may arise, depending on the diagnosis.

Conventional Treatment

Antibiotics are the treatment of choice for pelvic inflammatory disease. Other causes of pelvic pain are medicated accordingly.

What to Expect from Homeopathic Treatment

It is definitely worth treating pelvic pain homeopathically, although it is essential to establish a correct diagnosis. If the PID is a result of an untreated sexually transmitted disease, appropriate drugs should be taken first, followed by homeopathic treatment. Even when emergency medical care is required, such as in the case of an ectopic pregnancy, I have found homeopathy to work effectively and nearly immediately to relieve pain while the woman is transported to the hospital.

Naturopathic Suggestions to Complement Homeopathic Care

The recommendations depend entirely on the diagnosis, but here are some general guidelines.

- Eat a diet high in whole grains, fresh fruits, vegetables, and fiber.
- Drink at least six glasses of water a day.
- Minimize or avoid red meat and dairy products.
- If you eat poultry, make sure it's free of hormones and antibiotics.
- Avoid caffeine.
- Avoid or minimize alcohol.
- Do not smoke.
- Take a daily, high-quality megamultivitamin and mineral supplement including 300 milligrams of magnesium citrate malate.
- Take 1,200 milligrams a day of calcium citrate or, preferably, 600 milligrams a day of calcium citrate malate.
- If you have to take antibiotics, be sure to start taking acidophilus as soon as you finish. If you are highly prone to yeast infections as a result of antibiotics, there is another product I use, called Sacro-B, which is the only antibiotic-resistant form of acidophilus that I know of and can be used while you are on antibiotics.
- Packs in the form of ice, castor oil, or ginger can help relieve acute abdominal or pelvic pain.

PMS (Severe)

Kelly's Story

"My whole life changed from my first appointment with Judyth! Since the beginning of my menstrual cycle, at thirteen years of age, I have suffered. And, as the years went on, my PMS and endometriosis only increased in intensity and duration until I first saw her when I was twenty-eight.

"My periods began as heavy and lengthy, lasting five to seven full days. I struggled with backaches, bloating, severe irritability and anger, and unreasonable jealousy in any relationship in which I might be involved. In my younger years, these symptoms would creep up on me the week before; however, as I got older, they lasted ten days before my period! To me, this meant that for about fifteen days out of every month I was mad, bloated, extremely jealous, and plagued by pain in my lower back.

"It felt like I was going to explode, but I mostly held in my feelings because my anger frightened me. I imagine that this contributed to my getting into drugs and alcohol around the age of thirteen and into anorexia and bulimia later in my teens. I wanted so much to avoid the pain of my parents' divorce as well as the pain of just growing up. My cycle only made it worse. So I just tried to numb out. Finally, when I was twenty-six, I went into treatment and now have behind me eleven years of sobriety.

"As the years passed, my PMS got worse and worse. The pain increased and even the alcohol could not squelch my anger. The ache in my back grew considerably worse, and I began to experience severe stabbing pains in my rectum, due to the spread of the endometrial tissue. I also had trouble becoming pregnant. My husband and I tried for one year before I got pregnant the first time, then I miscarried at thirteen weeks. We kept trying, and it took another five and a half years until we had our daughter.

"I was very lucky to have found homeopathy. All of my PMS symptoms, distressing as they were, evaporated after the first homeopathic medicine Judyth gave me. Even more astounding, I got pregnant just three months later and gave birth to my beautiful daughter. I call her my homeopathic miracle baby. A year ago I gave birth to a wonderful son.

"My life has been incredibly better since I began homeopathic care. I am much more balanced, which makes my husband very happy, too! Judyth treats both of my children, and homeopathy has even helped our dog. We have all benefited immensely. I will be forever grateful that my life was given back to me."

I have witnessed Kelly heal and grow so much since I first started seeing her as a patient eight years ago. Two medicines had a profound effect on her during that time. *Calcarea phosphorica* (calcium phosphate) dramatically relieved her terribly distressing PMS (irritability, impatience, "massive" water retention, breast soreness, and uterine heaviness), rectal pain and uterine pain during sex due to endometriosis, jealousy, sacral pain, and salt craving. Plus, she got pregnant three months after her first dose of homeopathic medicine.

The second medicine that has helped Kelly with nearly every symptom over the past three and a half years is *Theridion* (orange spider), prescribed primarily due to her exquisite sensitivity to noise and fear of spiders. It has helped her with occasional hormonal problems and palpitations and has allowed Kelly to sail through another pregnancy with flying colors.

Description

Premenstrual syndrome (PMS) is probably the most universal women's problem (neck and neck with hot flashes), affecting four out of every five women, and embraces just about any physical, mental, or emotional symptoms imaginable. In fact, well over one hundred symptoms have been attributed to PMS. Whatever symptoms you have the rest of the month can potentially flare up before your period. If you have the misfortune to have really severe PMS, your distress can last up to two weeks before you start to bleed and may even continue several days into the period. This can mean three difficult weeks out of every month.

Symptoms

Common physical symptoms: breast tenderness, headaches, constipation, gas, bloating, fatigue, food cravings and binges, pelvic pain or discomfort, water retention, joint pain, herpes, acne, hives, back pain, heart palpitations, insomnia, clumsiness and accident proneness, hemorrhoids, ups and downs regarding sex drive, urinary problems, and others, including an exacerbation of whatever bothers you the rest of the month. Common mental and emotional symptoms: irritability, rage, mood swings, weepiness, depression, anxiety, confusion, indecision, and insecurity.

There may or may not be a predisposing cause other than hormonal changes. Some patients tell me their PMS is worse (or better) after deliveries, miscarriages, abortions, using birth control pills or injections, or having their tubes tied. Some studies link increased consumption of dairy products, caffeine, refined sugar, high estrogen and low progesterone levels, and excess body weight to PMS, as well as low levels of magnesium, vitamins C and E, and selenium.[5]

Complications

Premenstrual anger can, in rare cases, lead to suicidal or homicidal rage.

Conventional Treatment

It varies according to the symptoms and can include anti-anxiety or antidepressant medications, hormones, or other medications, depending on the particular symptoms.

What to Expect from Homeopathic Treatment

I have found homeopathy to be extremely effective for PMS, regardless of the specific symptoms, what caused it, or how long you have had it.

Naturopathic Suggestions to Complement Homeopathic Care

- Eat a diet high in whole grains, fresh fruits, vegetables (preferably organic), and fiber.
- Minimize or avoid red meat and dairy products.
- If you eat poultry, make sure it's free of hormones and antibiotics.
- Avoid caffeine.
- Avoid or minimize alcohol.
- Do not smoke.
- Take evening primrose, black currant, or borage oil capsules.
- Take one tablespoon of ground flaxseeds or flaxseed oil a day.
- Eat plenty of soy.
- Take a daily, high-quality megamultivitamin and mineral supplement including vitamin E, 400 to 800 IU; and vitamin C, 1,000 to 2,000 milligrams.
- Take 1,200 milligrams a day of calcium citrate or, preferably, 600 milligrams a day of calcium citrate malate.
- Take magnesium citrate malate, 300 milligrams a day.
- Lipotropic factors, particularly in combination with liver herbs such as dandelion root and milk thistle, can help the liver break down estrogen.
- Use natural progesterone cream from ovulation until the onset of your period.
- Herbs such as chaste tree and dong quai, either alone or in vitamin and mineral formulas, can be very helpful.
- Embark on a regular program of aerobic exercise for at least twenty minutes three times a week.
- Do yoga exercises specifically to tone the female organs.

Postpartum Depression (Severe)

Melissa's Story

Melissa is an easygoing, tell-it-like-it-is woman who has responded consistently well to homeopathy. You will have a chance to read more about her in the pregnancy section, which follows. Melissa was quite surprised at the toll her first pregnancy took on her. The excess weight and exhaustion left her drained of energy and enthusiasm. Her optimism went out the window and she became preoccupied with how she would get everything done. While Melissa usually had a healthy sexual appetite, the idea of sex now "repulsed" her. She described herself as "naggier" and "nitpickier" and was tired of nursing her baby. "Nothing makes me happy. I'm not me. I've become a real prude."

Sepia (cuttlefish ink), thankfully, turned her back into her normal congenial self. In fact, she felt much better within half an hour. She was thrilled, as, understandably, was her husband. Melissa fell into a slump shortly after the birth of her second child. Again, a dose of *Sepia* came to the rescue, restoring her energy, empathy, and libido.

Description
Severe postpartum depression is experiencing regret, sadness, or despair that begins immediately after the birth of your child. It can last for weeks to months and can put a terrific strain on caring for your newborn, as well on your primary relationship with any other young children you may have.

Symptoms
Postpartum depression, when it is extreme, can entail profound feelings of depression, even with thoughts of suicide or an aversion to, or violent impulses directed toward, the newborn.

Complications
In rare cases, postpartum depression is so severe that the mother seeks to abandon or hurt the child.

Conventional Treatment
Antidepressants may be recommended for severe postpartum depression, although there are concerns since most drugs can pass through breast milk to the nursing infant.

What to Expect from Homeopathic Treatment
Homeopathy can relieve postpartum depression quickly and effectively in most cases.

Naturopathic Suggestions to Complement Homeopathic Care
• Eat well for both of you, since you will be nursing your baby frequently. Eat lots of whole grains, organic fresh fruits and vegetables, fiber, and plenty of protein to keep up your energy.
• Drink at least six glasses of water a day.

- Avoid alcohol, caffeine, smoking, and excess sugar.
- Continue taking your prenatal vitamin/mineral as long as you are actively breastfeeding our baby. Make sure it contains 1,200 milligrams of calcium and 600 milligrams of magnesium, as well as at least 50 milligrams of B vitamins.
- If your postpartum depression is severe, get help.
- Continue nursing your baby.
- Be honest with your partner about your feelings.
- Get help taking care of the baby and other kids, if you have them.
- Talk with other moms who are going through or have survived postpartum depression.
- Nurture yourself with massages, flowers, soothing music, special treats, or whatever else makes you feel happy.
- Eat well, exercise, and relax.

Pregnancy-Related Problems

Melissa's Story

"I can say that I originally turned to homeopathy nine years ago, in my early twenties, for relief of stomach/ulcer/stress problems. Short of taking lots of antacids (which I HATE and can't really take well because they are PILLS), nothing had helped. Judyth's placing me on a constitutional homeopathic medicine changed my life by ridding me of my gastrointestinal problems, which I had resigned myself to face for the rest of my life. Thinking back, I realize that I've used homeopathy for a long time.

"Subsequent treatments included medicines for bleeding between periods, anger, hemorrhoids, and odd rashes. Homeopathy—and Dr. Reichenberg-Ullman—saw me through two pregnancies, including a degree of postpartum depression that was MUCH improved with a new homeopathic medicine.

"My strong constitutional health, and that of my two daughters, is based, I believe, on all of us being treated with homeopathy on an ongoing basis. My own inability to take pills or to stomach strong, allopathic medicines made me a homeopathic follower for life."

Melissa has relied on homeopathy to keep herself healthy since she started seeing me at twenty-four. My husband and I even attended her wedding! Melissa is an earthy, good-natured woman with a tendency toward fatigue, forgetfulness, hip pain, heartburn, genital herpes, hemorrhoids, and fear of heights; thus, *Calcarea carbonica* (calcium carbonate) has helped her for many years.

During Melissa's first pregnancy, she came to see me at fourteen weeks, due to a great deal of stomach acidity. She found that she gagged easily and all she wanted to eat were grapefruit and cold foods. One dose of *Veratrum album* (white hellebore) took care of the problem and she went on to deliver a robust and healthy little girl.

A year and a half later, she again showed up at my office seven weeks' pregnant, this time suffering from morning sickness and some heartburn. All she wanted was ice cold water, along with pickles and olives. *Veratrum album* once more rapidly relieved the problem.

 ### Description
Pregnancy lasts from the time you conceive until the time you deliver your baby.

 ### Symptoms
Breast tenderness and swelling and fatigue will likely be your first indicators of pregnancy. Morning sickness during your first trimester is common. From there, a myriad of symptoms or smooth sailing can follow. The most common include morning sickness, fatigue, back or joint pain, hypoglycemia, constipation, gas, heartburn, swelling, and moods varying from elation to sadness or indifference. The hormonal fluctuations that come with pregnancy can make you feel unpredictable and full of surprises—as if you don't even know yourself any more. The emotional ups and downs may last until you have delivered your baby or even longer.

 ### Complications
Too many complications are associated with pregnancy to mention them all, but some of the more typical are spotting or bleeding, miscarriage, placental problems, genital herpes, preeclampsia, toxemia, and difficult positioning of your baby in utero.

 ### Conventional Treatment
Problems are treated as they arise. It is common knowledge that many drugs can pass through the placenta, so most physicians are justifiably concerned about prescribing medications during pregnancy.

 ### What to Expect from Homeopathic Treatment
Not only do you not have to worry about doing any damage to your baby by taking homeopathic medicines during your pregnancy, but you will actually

do him a huge favor. Coming into balance yourself will allow you to deliver a healthier, happier baby. It appears that your being treated before the baby's birth may remove predispositions that he could otherwise inherit from you. The only way you can improve upon being treated homeopathically during your pregnancy is by doing so even earlier—prior to conceiving or, if you happen to have a very knowledgeable and alternatively minded mother, before *she* conceived you. You get the picture: the earlier, the better. Your receiving homeopathic care during your pregnancy can only help your baby.

Naturopathic Suggestions to Complement Homeopathic Care

- Eat exceptionally well for you and your growing baby.
- Eat a diet high in whole grains and fiber.
- Make sure you get about 75 grams of protein a day (that includes soy, eggs, dairy products, fish, and red meat).
- Eat lots of fresh fruits and vegetables.
- Now, more than ever, eat organic produce and make sure any animal proteins are free of hormones and antibiotics.
- Avoid pesticides and any household products that may be toxic.
- Take a high-quality prenatal vitamin and mineral with plenty of B vitamins, iron, folic acid, vitamin K, and calcium-magnesium.
- Red raspberry tea taken throughout the pregnancy can tone the uterus and make your delivery easier.
- Some herbs said to help prevent miscarriage are nettle, wild yam, and false unicorn.
- Surround yourself with a soothing, uplifting environment and a circle of support.
- Take time to create your ideal delivery, find a birthing team (this can include a doctor, midwife, coach, doula, and family members that you trust), make a birth plan, then take it as it comes.
- Cherish your intimacy and privacy with your partner because everything will be different in many ways after your baby is born.

Sexual Abuse

Meg's Story

"To give you an idea of what homeopathy has done for me, it is necessary to understand a bit of my background. Like many others, I had a sample, while growing up, of all of the types of abuse, from sexual to emotional, that a girl can experience right in her own seemingly normal and loving middle-class home, and, while I'm sure that experience has certainly shaped the unhealthy aspects of my personality, a large part of myself has always been, right from the beginning, rather inspired by and connected to life. Later on, though, during large segments of my life, keeping that in any kind of perspective at all was a tremendous challenge. In my thirties, there were definitely times when any ability to maintain insight and clarity was completely obscured.

"Fourteen years ago, after a night devoted to helping me through a rather difficult and terrifying asthma attack, a friend took me to her homeopath. My physical symptoms at that time ranged from chronic asthma to very out-of-control vertigo and hypoglycemia, as well as a stubborn case of tendinitis in my right arm. Many attendant emotional and mental symptoms also made it very difficult for me to hold a job, think clearly, talk to people, make friends, and express myself either verbally or in writing. All of these disabling problems led to my feeling extreme isolation, alienation, and imprisonment, with no choice but to mistakenly regard myself as gradually becoming mentally ill. But I could remember better days. My life had slowly and unarguably changed, so that by that time I hardly resembled the bright, young college student of ten years earlier who had felt so inspired and passionate about poetry, philosophy, and literature. Where did she go?

"Today I am a different woman. For a large part, most of the symptoms from which I initially suffered are pretty much gone, if not at least under control. I have a much clearer sense of self, feel worlds better about myself as a person and a woman, am in a happy relationship, and moved to a place where I really enjoy living. I feel happier and healthier than I have in many years. Even though I live quite far from Judyth, I still connect with her when I need to and she sends me a medicine.

"I've worked with Judyth for nine years. In the last analysis, I think that homeopathy has made it possible for me to come into alignment with my essential healthy self. It continues to do so today, bringing me clarity and control over my life and laying the groundwork for powerful changes in the sense of further personal growth and development, as well as giving me a broader perspective into my own life and life in general."

Seeing Meg give birth to the fullness of her being has been a great joy for me. When I first met her ten years ago, she was so shy and uneasy about sharing her innermost feelings that we could only have fifteen-minute appointments. Now, when the appointments are short, it is only because she lives on another continent and is trying to economize.

Meg's hypoglycemia was quite debilitating, leaving her disoriented and floaty. She felt smothered by her allergies, which turned into frightening asthma attacks. Her digestion was in quite a state of disorder at the beginning of treatment, with frequent belching, loose stools, and a sense of having a hole in her stomach. Her periods were too frequent and her memory faulty. But mostly, Meg's extreme self-consciousness, shyness, and introspection stood in the way of her becoming all she could be.

It took a number of years for me, as well as for Meg herself, to get to the bottom of why she held herself back so. It was a direct result of abuse during childhood, which she had not known how to process. She had ended up doubting herself and feeling unable to get close to anyone.

Meg is literally a different woman. The medicine that helped her for the first year was *Lycopodium* (club moss), but the one that has made a truly profound difference in her body and psyche over the past six years is *Lac caninum* (dog's milk). It is a wonderful medicine for women who feel put down and inadequate, much like the bottom dog in a pack. Her floaty feeling during the hypoglycemia, plus her frequent dreams of snakes and her self-consciousness, are confirmations of the medicine.

Meg is now in a healthy and happy relationship with another woman—her transformation has been one of the more remarkable ones I have seen in my practice.

Description

Sexual abuse covers a range of behaviors, from verbal innuendos to exposure, touching the breasts and genital organs, sodomy, cunnilingus, fellatio, and penetration. Though sexual abuse, either during childhood or adulthood, is far more widely recognized than when I trained as a psychiatric social worker in the 1970s, many more cases go unreported than those that are. If someone were to ask me to name the one most devastating experience that I find over and over again in working with women, it is unquestionably sexual abuse. The amount of pain, shame, dysfunction, and devastation that can result, sometimes lifelong, is heartwrenching.

Symptoms

Physical symptoms vary tremendously but can include all kinds of bladder and gynecological complaints and just about any other complaint that started right after or within a few years of the abuse, or even later, such as when memories are recovered. Psychological symptoms are also myriad. Some of the most common are low self-esteem, a history of unsatisfactory relationships, eating disorders, depression, anxiety, panic disorder, and multiple personality (dissociative identity) disorder.

Complications

A serious physical concern is sexually transmitted diseases. Psychologically, the loss of innocence and the subsequent shame and terror are as great as any physical complication and can be detrimental to future intimate relationships.

Conventional Treatment

Treatment ranges from immediate post-rape intervention to address the possibility of pregnancy and sexually transmitted diseases, to years of medication and psychotherapy as needed.

What to Expect from Homeopathic Treatment

Homeopathy can be a terrific help to women who have experienced sexual abuse at any time in their lives, and it can often help them to dramatically turn their lives around for the better.

Naturopathic Suggestions to Complement Homeopathic Care

- Take care of your body through diet, nutritional supplements, and exercise.
- Surround yourself with people who are gentle when you need to be treated with TLC and who truly care about you.
- Love yourself and accept love from others, no matter what you have been through.
- Get help from a competent and experienced psychotherapist or hypnotherapist whom you trust. Countless types of therapy can be beneficial.
- As you understand yourself better and gain more tools to deal with what happened to you, you will be more able to choose loving, caring, and safe intimate relationships in the future.
- Understand that recovery from sexual abuse takes time and happens in stages and that memories may continue to surface for years.
- Protect yourself in whatever way you need to from your abuser.

Uterine Fibroids

Caroline's Story

"My gynecologist diagnosed me with uterine fibroids, which, he advised me, were steadily growing. He counseled me that there was really nothing short of a hysterectomy that would help. The sooner, he recommended, the better. If I could only make it to menopause, he added, it was likely that my fibroids would shrink and the symptoms would improve. But, being only forty at the time, that was ten years of biding time! At least, I was fortunate that cancer was not causing my symptoms and that I had some time to find another solution.

"I felt very strongly that surgery was not the only answer, but I didn't know where to turn. A second gynecologist, whom I consulted for a second opinion, gave me identical advice except that he urged me to have a hysterectomy within two months at the latest. He also added that I might as well have my ovaries removed along with my uterus because he'd probably have to take them out sooner or later.

"My aunt had died of cancer directly related to taking hormone-replacement therapy and I had no desire to give up my hormone-producing organs if there was a way to save them. My goal was to avoid what I considered to be unnecessary surgery and to somehow find a way to make my fibroids shrink, or at least not to get any larger. After all, some imbalance caused them to grow, so I must be able to do something to bring myself back into balance. But what? Neither doctor offered any explanation as to why they grew and even less about treatment options.

"I have always leaned toward natural remedies and decided to try everything I could before submitting to surgery. I found Dr. Reichenberg-Ullman, and, after taking my health history and interviewing me extensively about many aspects of my life, she prescribed a homeopathic medicine.

"Within my next menstrual cycle, I noticed improvement in all symptoms. Homeopathy also cleared up two other chronic problems: eczema on my face and constipation. Many other things in my life improved as well, as a direct result of the homeopathic treatment, including my finding the courage to go back to school to pursue a more fulfilling career and finding my dream house and husband. Homeopathy truly does work on all levels to bring one's life closer to balance.

"I thank Dr. Reichenberg-Ullman for saving my organs from the surgeon's scalpel and bettering my life overall."

The medicine *Silica* (flint) has been a gift to Caroline for the past five years. It is an excellent medicine for fibroids in women who are reserved, refined, quiet, and just plain nice, which is what people who know Caroline say about her. Women needing *Silica*, like Caroline, are chilly and tend to have performance anxiety. There is also a pronounced tendency toward constipation.

The medicine was very helpful for Caroline's heavy periods and clotting, facial eczema, breast tenderness, and premenstrual headaches. Her fibroids have been kept at bay for five years and, now that she is menopausal, will likely decrease in size so as not to be a problem. During that period of time, she has found a loving husband, a new career that she loves, and a greater sense of self-confidence.

Description

Uterine fibroids (leiomyomas or myomas) are benign growths of muscle tissue in the uterus. Fibroids are extremely common, occurring in 20 to 25 percent of women by age forty and in 50 percent of women in general and are the most common cause of major surgery in women.[6] Although fibroids are almost always benign, they do pose a risk factor for uterine cancer and it appears that both problems, as in a number of other women's conditions, are mediated by high estrogen levels. Uterine fibroids generally resolve on their own once you reach menopause.

Symptoms

Women with fibroids often have no symptoms at all, but uterine heaviness, bloating, discomfort, or pain, excessive or irregular bleeding, pain with intercourse, and urinary frequency are the most typical symptoms.

Complications

Rarely, in about 1 percent of cases, fibroids are malignant. The complications that are most likely to result in a hysterectomy are profuse bleeding and urinary symptoms resulting from the fibroid pressing against the bladder. Because the growth of fibroids is estrogen-mediated, fibroids can enlarge considerably in pregnancy, sometimes, depending on size and position, endangering the fetus. Rarely, the fibroid can press on the ureter, causing kidney damage.

Conventional Treatment

By far the most common solution that orthodox medicine offers for uterine fibroids is hysterectomy, either total or partial. (I urge you to keep your ovaries unless there is some compelling reason not to do so.) Another option is myomectomy (removal of only the fibroid), but it is not always effective over the long run and very few surgeons are willing to do it.

What to Expect from Homeopathic Treatment

Nearly all of my patients with fibroids, with the exception of only a few, have made it to menopause with their uteruses intact. I have not found the fibroids to shrink (except in one case) or disappear, but they rarely grow and do not require invasive interventions. Homeopathy usually takes care of the discomfort, bleeding, and urinary problems quite nicely.

Naturopathic Suggestions to Complement Homeopathic Care

- Eat a diet high in whole grains, fresh fruits, vegetables (preferably organic), and fiber.
- Drink at least six glasses of water a day.
- Avoid red meat and dairy products.
- Avoid caffeine.
- Avoid or minimize alcohol.
- Do not smoke.
- Take evening primrose, black currant, or borage oil capsules.
- Take one tablespoon of ground flaxseeds or flaxseed oil a day.
- Eat plenty of soy.
- Take a daily, high-quality megamultivitamin and mineral supplement including vitamin E, 400 to 800 IU.
- Take 1,200 milligrams a day of calcium citrate or, preferably, 600 milligrams a day of calcium citrate malate.
- Take magnesium citrate malate, 300 milligrams a day.
- Lipotropic factors, particularly in combination with liver herbs such as dandelion root and milk thistle, can help the liver break down estrogen and are an essential component of my fibroid protocol.
- Use natural progesterone cream throughout the month except during your period.
- Naturopathic physicians who do not use homeopathy use herbal formulas for uterine fibroids.
- Embark on a regular program of aerobic exercise for at least twenty minutes, three times a week.
- Do yoga exercises that specifically tone the female organs.

Vaginal Infections (Recurrent)

Nancy's Story

"After laparoscopic surgery to remove an ovarian cyst, during which that ovary and scar tissue were also removed (probably due to an improperly treated infection in the past), I developed painful and recurring vaginitis. Nothing seemed to get rid of it. My uterus felt so swollen that my insides put pressure on the nerves in my back and down my legs. I didn't know what was due to the infection, what was due to surgery, and what I had to live with. I was miserable. My gynecologist prescribed one antibiotic after another. The infection kept returning. This went on for a whole year. The antibiotics caused their own set of symptoms and I refused to continue taking them.

"I have used homeopathy symptomatically for years for myself and my dogs, cats, and friends with great success to treat injuries, colds, grief, and so forth. There are no homeopaths whom I trust where I live and I was thrilled to learn that Dr. Reichenberg does phone consultations. Answering her questions took considerable self-examination, which was useful in itself.

"The medicine that she gave me started working quite dramatically eight days after I took it. I had a wonderful dream that night (I rarely remember my dreams) and more vivid dreams for weeks. The infection had been horrible, but that day it was gone entirely!

"My periods have gotten lighter and my PMS is much better, as far as out-of-control emotions and muscle tension. In general, I feel happier.

"I have antidoted my medicine twice now—once in a hotel, breathing strong dry cleaning fumes from the room next door. I checked out in a hurry! The infection started to return afterward, but after a few days the homeopathic medicine took hold again and the infection disappeared. More recently, I used a strong cleanser called Simple Green, and it totally wiped out the homeopathic medicine. The dose that I took afterward isn't working as effectively as before, so I will probably need a higher one soon.

"I am so impressed that a skilled homeopath could pick the perfect remedy for me. I have total confidence in homeopathy keeping me infection-free when nothing else could, and allowing me to attain a state of greater health, physically and emotionally."

Nancy had suffered from a copious vaginal discharge since she was a teenager, which was diagnosed in recent years as a bacterial vaginal infection. More recently, she was troubled by uterine swelling that became worse from any emotional upset, and spotting between periods. A year before beginning homeopathic treatment, Nancy had her left ovary and fallopian tube removed, due to a cyst. At that time the surgeon also discovered a small amount of endometriosis. Her periods continued to be heavy and clotted, and she complained of a searing pain in her uterus during the second half of her period, as if her skin were being ripped off.

Nancy's internal script was one of feeling not good enough and thinking that there was something wrong with her. She felt criticized by her partner when he had no intention of doing so, which came from her oversensitivity as a little girl. She used to cry if her mother even looked cross-eyed at her. When depressed, Nancy sunk into a horrible, cavernous, bottomless abyss.

Nancy's vaginitis vanished after she took *Thuja* (arbor vitae), a medicine that can be quite helpful for vaginal discharge, growths such as cysts and tumors, and a negative feeling about oneself. Her periods have been lighter, her bloating is gone, and she feels happier and more balanced emotionally.

Janey's Story

"Strep throats, bronchitis, and yeast infections plagued my growing-up years. As an adult, five years ago, I got a horrendous cold that turned into laryngitis, bronchitis, and eventually asthma that would not go away. Doctors gave me steroids and multiple inhalers. They kept telling me I would be off the drugs in a month, but that didn't happen.

"The drugs messed with my body and started causing additional challenges like vaginal yeast infections. The itch was horrible, like one thousand fleas living in, around, and outside my vagina, having the party of their lives! Pure torture is the best way to describe it. My days were consumed by symptoms that ravaged my breathing, my vagina, and my self-esteem. Life was completely out of control and I was my own victim.

"Ultimately, I found Judyth. Homeopathy was all a very foreign process to me, yet it made perfect sense. For the first time in my life, all aspects of me, physical, emotional, and spiritual, were addressed, rather than just my asthma and yeast infections. I have been asthma-free for four years, the yeast infections are no longer a problem, and I'm proud to say that my quality of life, attitude, and self-esteem have skyrocketed."

Janey is one of my most fun patients—a live wire, enthusiastic and vivacious. I have seen her now for six years. Her initial state was one of being overwhelmed and feeling controlled by the chaos that swirled around her. Janey worried entirely too much about all kinds of things, especially her husband, family, finances, and her health. Part of her was stuck in the despondency and overconcern. Another part was upbeat and positive and tried to tell herself to let go and be happy. Janey's oldest sister had suffered from ovarian cancer.

Janey's main women's complaints were, first, vaginal itching that drove her crazy, so much so that she couldn't stop herself from scratching, and second, herpes outbreaks that wouldn't quit. She was overcome with desperation when the vaginitis hit her. She also experienced bleeding in between her periods.

Janey tended to attract crises into her life, which she somehow managed to deal with quite effectively. Yet, during each crisis, her predominant feeling was of being out of control. Her worrying ran her life.

The homeopathic medicine that had the biggest impact on Janey was *Argentum ni-tricum* (silver nitrate). This medicine is helpful for anxious, excitable, outgoing women who are great crisis managers and feel very uneasy when things are out of control. It has taken care of the vaginitis, reduced the herpes outbreaks to a minimum (except when the medicine was antidoted), eliminated the bleeding between periods, and helped a variety of other physical problems as well. She is much calmer and less preoccupied and is happy in a demanding job that creates enough crises for her not to have to generate so many at home.

One of the annoying side effects of peri- and postmenopause can be atrophic vaginitis, a thinning of the vaginal tissue due to lack of estrogen, which can cause pain and discomfort and make sex uncomfortable or out of the question.

Robin's Story

"I am a fifty-one-year-old woman who has experienced perimenopausal symptoms for five years or so. Except for excessive menstrual bleeding (probably from fibroids) that was treated well with Prometrium (oral micronized progesterone) and some occasional 'warm flushes' at night, I had no troublesome symptoms.

"Then, a few years ago, I encountered real problems with vaginal atrophy. My vaginal tissues were so dry and fragile that they could become bruised and sore with sex and highly susceptible to yeast infections. I didn't take kindly to these limitations on what had been a great sexual relationship with my husband.

"My gynecologist had long pressured me to take HRT (hormone-replacement therapy) to reduce my risk of osteoporosis and heart disease, despite the fact that I had a very, very low risk for either. Then he played his trump card: Estrogen would restore the altered pH of my vagina and cure my yeast infections and vaginal dryness.

"Admittedly motivated by sex, I started taking oral estradiol. It seemed to work at first, but then I began to experience itching, bruising, dryness, and one or two yeast infections a month. I exhibited some signs of too much estrogen, so he cut the daily dosage in half, to 0.5 mg, but the vaginal problems did not improve.

"At this point, I had the option of taking antifungal medication for several months and/or adding a messy vaginal estradiol cream to the mix. I decided to try another tactic entirely. My husband reminded me that several years earlier a constitutional homeopathic medicine had cleared up my yeast infections for about a year. I felt as if conventional medicine wouldn't help to balance the alkalinity/acidity of my vagina, so I called Judyth.

"At first, I experienced an odd sense of the presence of my uterus. It felt like a weight for a few days. I chalked the sensation up to "homeopathic weirdness." Within a week my vaginal problems had disappeared. No more yeast infections and

I've been able to resume the sex life I had before. I do have to avoid Chap Stick, Vicks, and Pine-Sol, but my husband says he'll gladly clean the toilets forever if this medicine continues to work." (Note: Robin has since stopped the hormone replacement because of its potential to aggravate the fibroids and is doing fine.)

Compared to most of us, Robin had no particular unresolved emotional issues. She had a good marriage and family, a strong spiritual life, a happy family of origin, an active sex life, and lots of friends. No matter how much I investigated Robin's symptoms and overall picture, she just needed help with her atrophic vaginitis, which was, in and of itself, severe. Her labia was dry, hot, burning, and itchy. Sex was uncomfortable, to say the least. She also had uterine fibroids, a history of heavy menstrual bleeding, and a cervical polyp that had been removed, as well as an IUD-induced pelvic inflammatory disease.

Fortunately, it only took one medicine, *Thuja* (arbor vitae), to end Robin's nagging vaginal irritation. It is an excellent medicine for fragile tissue of the labia and vagina as well as for fibroids and polyps. Given her overall level of health, Robin will need infrequent homeopathic visits.

Description

Chronic vaginitis can be triggered by a viral, bacterial, trichomonal, or yeast infection; sexual contact; douching; or other irritants such as diaphragms, cervical caps, or menstrual sponges. Atrophic vaginitis, resulting from a decrease in estrogen levels, is a quite common cause of chronic infections, often in combination with yeast, in postmenopausal women.

Symptoms

Vaginal discharge, of varying thickness or thinness, odorless or offensive, bland or acrid, is often the main symptom. Irritation of the labia and vulva can create great distress in the form of swelling, rawness, discomfort, fragility, and pain. The vagina itself can also be very uncomfortable and painful.

Complications

Serious conditions such as gonorrhea, chlamydia, and HIV infections must be ruled out, though your vaginitis is most likely to be due to a yeast infection and, less often, to a bacterial infection or atrophic vaginitis. Atrophic vaginitis often coexists with yeast infections.

Conventional Treatment

Antifungal medications in the form of a cream or taken orally are most commonly prescribed.

What to Expect from Homeopathic Treatment

Homeopathy, sometimes in combination with other natural treatments, is very effective for chronic vaginal infections.

Naturopathic Suggestions to Complement Homeopathic Care

* Eat a diet high in whole grains, organic fruits and vegetables, and fiber.
* Drink at least six glasses of water a day.
* Avoid red meat and minimize other animal products.
* Eliminate caffeine, alcohol, and smoking.
* Cut out or decrease sweets, fruit juice, and dried fruits if you have chronic yeast infections.
* Avoid nylon underpants, pantyhose, and tightly fitting pants.
* Eliminate diaphragms, cervical caps, and menstrual sponges if they trigger your infections.
* Practice safe sex. For persistent, recurrent infections, consider condoms.
* Eat unsweetened yogurt on a regular basis.
* Boric acid and acidophilus suppositories are often at least palliatively effective. Insert one capsule of boric acid powder vaginally in the morning and one capsule of acidophilus at bedtime for five days. Stop during your period.
* Douche with one tablespoon of white vinegar in a pint of warm water daily for five days. Insert one tablespoon of unsweetened, live-culture yogurt after each douche.
* Occasionally, one tablespoon of baking soda in a quart of warm water works better as a douche than do acidifying treatments such as vinegar or boric acid.
* If the vaginitis is only on the labia and vulva, and is caused by yeast, apply a preparation of half vinegar and half water topically.
* Some women insert a clove of garlic, wrapped in cheesecloth or gauze, vaginally for yeast infections.
* If there is rawness externally *not* due to yeast, *Calendula* cream topically can be helpful.
* Various lubricants, including K-Y Jelly, SYLK, and Creme de la Femme can increase vaginal moisture and make sex much more enjoyable.
* Insert vitamin E suppositories into the vagina for atrophic vaginitis.
* *Calendula,* vitamin A, or herbal vaginal suppositories can be soothing.

Vaginismus

Patty's Story

Patty begged off for not being a writer and asked me to share her story for her. The main two problems that brought Patty to see me, when she was thirty-one, were horrible menstrual cramps since the age of twelve and vaginismus. She also suffered from high blood pressure and PMS. Patty's cramps were so severe around menarche that she couldn't even walk! They forced her to stay home from school each month during the incapacitating part of her period. Her doctors put her on birth control pills at age fourteen, but she lost ten pounds, had frightening nightmares about skeletons with black hoods, and cried all the time. The weight loss, weeping, and nightmares went away within three months of discontinuing the pill, but the cramps came back. Patty had tried "every anti-inflammatory on the market" and even resorted to the pill again from age eighteen to twenty-two, then quit.

Unmedicated, she experienced burning, tearing pain as if someone had run a knife with a dull, serrated blade back and forth across her abdomen. It felt as if her uterus weighed fifty pounds during this time. Her cramps were often accompanied by right-sided sciatica. She also complained of ovarian pain at ovulation, fibrocystic breasts, and left-sided headaches on waking. During her PMS, things that normally wouldn't bother Patty really bugged her. She found herself yelling in traffic and thinking, "Why don't you hurry up?" around all the slugs at her office.

Just as debilitating as Patty's cramps was her vaginismus, probably resulting from scar tissue after a surgery at age nineteen. Sex was terribly painful. Patty wondered if there was some connection between her vaginismus and other hormonal problems to sexual abuse by a neighbor when she was five years old, which she had not revealed to anyone.

It is five years since Patty started seeing me for homeopathy and she is better in all ways. The medicine that has helped her is *Lachesis* (bushmaster snake). She also went to a sex therapist who educated her about vaginismus and gave her a series of vaginal dilators of graduated sizes.

The *Lachesis* normalized Patty's blood pressure, dramatically improved her headaches and vaginismus (along with the dilators and a wonderful new marriage), breast cysts, and premenstrual anger, as well as helping her with her periods. She and her new husband hope to become pregnant in the near future.

Description
An involuntary spasm of the vagina.

Symptoms
Vaginal pain during sex or a speculum exam can be extreme.

Complications
Inability to engage in intercourse or to have pelvic examinations.

Conventional Treatment
The graduated dilation technique is the most common treatment.

What to Expect from Homeopathic Treatment
Homeopathy can be effective for vaginismus, often in conjunction with therapy.

Naturopathic Suggestions to Complement Homeopathic Care
• Create an optimal program of a natural foods diet, nutritional supplements, a health enhancing lifestyle, and loving relationships.
• Undergo psychotherapy to uncover and resolve any underlying blocks, such as sexual abuse, unhappy past intimate relationships, or damaging messages from your parents about sex.
• Try counseling with your partner, preferably with a sex therapist or psychotherapist who is experienced in helping people with sexual problems.
• Find a partner who is gentle, loving, and understanding; does not pressure you about sex; and is willing to give you time.
• Learn to find other ways besides penetration to satisfy yourself and your partner, at least until you find intercourse comfortable.

PART FOUR

Materia Medica

CHAPTER **14**

Fifty Homeopathic Medicines for Women's Acute Self-Care

Following are fifty homeopathic medicines that I believe you will find most helpful for treating yourself, and the same ones, consequently, that I have included in the Women's Self-Care Medicine Kit, which is a companion to this book. You may need other medicines, but, if you have these medicines with you and suffer from one of the conditions included in the self-care section of this book, the chances are high that you will find a medicine that is of benefit.

The symptoms I have put in **bold** font are those that are the most prominent for self-prescribing the indicated medicine. You should, therefore, give them more weight, or importance, when deciding which medicine to choose. In other words, if you have mastitis of your right breast, it is likely, from the bold type, that *Phytolacca* will be of greater benefit than *Magnesia phosphorica,* also a medicine that favors the right side but that is not well-indicated for glandular swellings. I have tried to organize this information in a way that you will find extremely user-friendly.

Aconite (Monkshood)

Key Symptoms
Ailments from fright or shock
Extreme anxiety, restlessness, and excitability
Fear that you will die
Symptoms come on suddenly

Mind
Claustrophobia
Fear of airplanes, crowds, earthquakes
Panic attacks
Afraid to be alone

Body
Profuse perspiration with anxiety
Rapid pulse

Breasts and Female Genitalia
Fear that you will die during labor
Screaming with pain
Your period stops because of a fear or shock
Threatened miscarriage after a fright

Worse
Chill

Better
Rest
Fresh air

Food and Drink
Very thirsty for cold drinks

Aesculus (Horse chestnut)

Key Symptoms
Hemorrhoids
Affected parts are purple
Puffiness and fullness

Mind
Confused
Sluggish

Body
Sensation of shooting pains in the rectum
Back pain or sciatica with hemorrhoids
Hemorrhoid pain long after bowel movements
Constipation

Breasts and Female Genitalia
Painful hemorrhoids during pregnancy
Hemorrhoids after childbirth

Worse
Morning on waking
Stooping after a bowel movement

Better
After the hemorrhoids bleed
Taking a bath

Food and Drink
Aversion to food in general

Apis mellifica (Honeybee)

Key Symptoms
Swelling
Redness and heat
Burning and stinging pain

Mind and Emotions
Busy as a bee
Protect your hive (family or home)
Jealous

Body
Right-sided symptoms
Swelling of eyes, face, throat, ovaries
Symptoms develop quickly and pains come suddenly

Breasts and Female Genitalia
Right ovarian cysts
Bladder infections with lots of swelling
Vaginal swelling better from cold packs

Worse
Problems from suppressing sexual desire
Heat

Better
Cold applications

Food and Drink
Lack of thirst

Arnica (Leopard's bane)

Key Symptoms
Trauma, injuries, falls, sprains, or strains
Bruising
Shock
Bleeding anywhere in the body
Before and after surgery

Mind
You refuse help
Insist that nothing is wrong

Body
Skin is black and blue following injury
Muscles are sore and achy
Sore, bruised feeling anywhere in the body

Breasts and Female Genitalia
Sore, bruised feeling after labor
Postpartum hemorrhage with shock
Threatened miscarriage after a fall or injury
Mastitis from an injury

Worse
Touch
Overexertion

Better
Lying down with the head low

Arsenicum album (Arsenic)

Key Symptoms
Tremendous anxiety
Fear of death
Restlessness
Burning pains anywhere in the body

Mind
Very anxious about your health
Fear of germs and contagion
Complain that you will not recover
Cranky and fastidious

Body
Weakness and loss of weight
Freezing cold

Symptoms are worse after midnight
Maddening pains

 Breasts and Female Genitalia
Burning pains in the ovary or breast
Putrid-smelling menses
Vaginal discharge comes instead of menstrual flow
Profuse, yellow, thick, burning vaginal discharge
Increased sexual desire during your period

 Worse
Midnight to 2 A.M.
Cold food or drinks

 Better
Heat
Warm drinks

 Food and Drink
Want to sip cold drinks frequently
Desire for milk

Belladonna (Deadly nightshade)

 Key Symptoms
Bright-red bleeding
Sunstroke or heat exhaustion
Sudden onset of symptoms
Extreme sensitivity to noise, light, and being jarred

 Mind
Sudden outbursts of anger
Vivacious, intense, and exuberant

Body
Right-sided symptoms
Throbbing pains
Symptoms are violent
Fullness and congestion

Breasts and Female Genitalia
Profuse, gushing, bright-red menstrual flow
Pelvic congestion
Mastitis with throbbing pain, heat, and red streaks
Sensation of organs falling out through the vagina

Worse
Touch
Being jarred
Afternoon, especially 3 P.M.
Exposure to sun

Better
Quiet, dark, rest
Bending backward in a semi-erect position

Food and Drink
Either great thirst for cold water or no thirst at all
Desire for lemons and lemonade

Bellis perennis (Daisy)

Key Symptoms
Muscle soreness
Sprains and bruises
Sore, bruised feeling in the pelvic area

Mind
Despair during pain
Don't know where you are

Body
Injuries in which the swelling persists
Injuries to pelvic organs

Breasts and Female Genitalia
Can't walk during pregnancy due to strain or injury of abdominal muscles
Bearing down sensation after childbirth
Uterine pain during pregnancy
Bleeding between periods after exertion

Worse
Injury
Touch
Cold bath, shower, or cold drinks
Becoming chilled after being overheated

Better
Continuing to move

Food and Drink
Desire for pickled food

Bryonia (Wild hops)

Key Symptoms
Worse from any motion
Very irritable
Parched
Extreme thirst for cold drinks

Mind
Longing to go home
Talk incessantly about your work
Fear of poverty

Body
Dryness of mucous membranes
Worse at 9 P.M.
Injuries or fractures that are worse from any movement

Breasts and Female Genitalia
Mastitis that is worse from even slight movement
Mastitis with hard, hot breasts
Uterine or ovarian pain that is worse from motion
Brown menstrual blood

Worse
Motion
Anger
Becoming overheated

Better
Pressure
Lying on the painful side
Wet and cloudy weather

Cactus grandifolia (Night-blooming cereus)

Key Symptoms
Squeezing pains like a vise
Heart feels alternately clutched and released
Congestion

Mind
You feel encaged
Dreams of falling

Body
Constriction, particularly of muscles
Feeling of an iron hand squeezing the heart
Bleeding with rapid clot formation

Breasts and Female Genitalia
Tightness of bladder, vagina, uterus
Period flows during the day and stops on lying down
Excruciating menstrual cramps
Vaginal spasms and constriction during sex

Worse
11:00 P.M.
Lying down
Exertion

Better
Fresh air
Rest

Food and Drink
Aversion to meat

Caladium (American arum)

Key Symptoms
Intense vaginal itching
Dryness of body parts
Problems from smoking

Mind
Apprehensive about your health
Think a lot about sex
Do not want to take medicine

Body
Want to remain still and not move
Very high or low sexual energy, combined with craving for tobacco
Coldness of various parts of the body

Breasts and Female Genitalia
Vaginal itching during pregnancy
Desire to masturbate with the itching
Uterine cramps at night

Worse
Cold drinks
Warm room

Better
Fresh air
Sweating

Food and Drink
Craving for tobacco

Calcarea carbonica (Calcium carbonate)

Key Symptoms
Overweight and sluggish
Worried about safety and security
Practical, down-to-earth
Illnesses from taking on too much responsibility

Mind
Independent
Obstinate
Overwhelmed
Fear of flying, heights, mice, insanity
Anxious about your health

Body
Symptoms that come on after exertion
Calf, foot, and thigh cramps

Profuse perspiration, especially on your head
Low thyroid

Breasts and Female Genitalia
Milky, burning, itchy vaginal discharge
Absence of periods
Heavy prolonged period, especially after exertion
Excessive production of watery milk that disagrees with your baby

Worse
Cold, damp weather
Exertion
Going uphill

Better
Staying warm
Dry weather
Rest

Food and Drink
Desire for eggs, sweets, and salt

Cantharis (Spanish fly)

Key Symptoms
Bladder infections, especially severe and of sudden onset
Burns of any kind
Burning pains

Mind
Frenzy
Restlessness
Distress on being touched or approached
Excessive sexual energy

Body
Violently acute bladder infection
Severe pain in the bladder or urethra at the beginning of or during urination
Bloody urine
Urine burning or scalding

Breasts and Female Genitalia
Heightened sexual desire during bladder infections
Constant urge to urinate
Urinary tract infection is aggravated by intercourse
Urine is passed one drop at a time

Worse
Urinating
Cold

Better
Warmth
Rest

Food and Drink
Desire for wine

Castor equi (Rudimentary thumbnail of the horse)

Key Symptoms
Nipples, nails, and bone problems
Cracked, sore nipples in nursing mothers
Breasts are sore and swollen

Mind
Dreams of your mother
Dreams of sick people
Laughing for no reason

Body

Nipples are so sensitive that clothing or being touched is unbearable
Nipples are cracked to the point of being ragged
Dry, painful nipples
Red areola

Breasts and Female Genitalia

Breast pain after delivery
Nipples raw from rubbing
Abscessed, ulcerated nipples

Worse

Nursing
Pressure from clothing

Better

Giving the breast a rest

Food and Drink

Desire for tobacco

Caulophyllum (Blue cohosh)

Key Symptoms

Erratic pains fly from place to place
Stalled labor
Pains are cramping, drawing, shooting
Neck is stiff and sore

Mind

Excitable
Worried, apprehensive
Irritable

Body
Rigid os
Atony of uterus
Weak or irregular labor pains
False labor

Breasts and Female Genitalia
Pricking, needlelike pains in cervix
Labor pains stop due to exhaustion or pain
Lengthy and exhausting labor
Uterine pain after delivery

Worse
Cold

Better
Being warm

Food and Drink
Worse from coffee

Chamomilla (Chamomile)

Key symptoms
Tremendous hypersensitivity to pain
Nasty and rude
Unbearable pain

Mind
Symptoms are worse from anger
Capricious
Your moods put off other people
Inconsolable

Body
Excruciating menstrual pain
Pain is so intense that you vomit
Green-colored diarrhea

Breasts and Female Genitalia
Menstrual pain after anger
Profuse, dark, clotted menses
Occasional gushing of bright-red blood
Menstrual pain extends down your thighs

Worse
Anger
Night
Lying in bed

Better
Menstrual pain relieved by heat and pressure
Cold applications

Food and Drink
Desire for cold water and sour drinks
Aversion to coffee

China (Peruvian bark)

Key Symptoms
Weakness from loss of body fluids
Periodic symptoms
Anemia
Face is pale

Mind
Daydreaming, full of ideas
Fantasies about doing great things

You feel picked on or persecuted
Fear of dogs

Body
Weakness and exhaustion after loss of body fluids
Symptoms come and go periodically
Anemia
Tremendous bloating

Breasts and Female Genitalia
Extreme exhaustion and weakness after labor or postpartum bleeding
Being touched during labor is intolerable
Oversensitive to noise during labor

Worse
Loss of fluids
Touch
Being jarred

Better
Hard pressure
Loosening clothes

Food and Drink
Desire for cherries

Cimicifuga (Black cohosh)

Key Symptoms
Cramping pains
Feel trapped
Nape of neck is very sensitive to drafts
Muscle soreness

Mind
Gloomy, as if enveloped in a black cloud
Feel trapped after your baby is born
Fear that you are going crazy
Sighing
Talkative, jump from one topic to another

Body
Stiffness and pain in neck, back, hips
Major menopausal medicine
Joint pains during menopause
Pains fly across the abdomen from side to side

Breasts and Female Genitalia
The more profuse the menstrual flow, the worse the symptoms
Labor pains that bring on fainting
Soreness and stiffness of whole body after labor
Shivers during the first stage of labor

Worse
Labor
Drafts

Better
Wrapping up
Holding on to your thighs

Food and Drink
Worse from alcohol
Desire for cold water

Cocculus (Indian cockle)

Key Symptoms
Motion sickness, airsickness, seasickness
Ailments from caring for others
Dehydration

Mind

Weakness after loss of sleep or caring for a loved one

Nervous exhaustion

Confusion and disorientation

Body

Dizziness worse from looking at moving objects or out the window of a moving vehicle

Nausea from dizziness

Nausea from thinking about or smelling food

Breasts and Female Genitalia

Periods are too early, too heavy, too frequent

Extreme weakness during your period

Gushing vaginal discharge

Hemorrhoids after menstrual pain

Worse

During your period

Loss of sleep

Traveling

Better

Sitting

Lying on your side

Food and Drink

Aversion to food

Coffea (Unroasted coffee)

Key Symptoms

Overstimulation, hypersensitivity, and hyperexcitability

Nervous agitation and restlessness

Unusual activity of body and mind

Exquisite sensitivity to pain
Hypersensitivity to noise, light, and touch

Mind
Overreaction to all emotions, even joy and surprise
Extreme nervous tension and anxiety
Abundance of ideas
Boundless energy to complete tasks

Body
Very low pain threshold
Terrible toothaches
Wide awake at 3 A.M. with mind full of thoughts
High sexual energy

Breasts and Female Genitalia
Periods come too early and last too long
Severe labor pains or uterine pain after delivery
Vaginal itch that you must scratch
Painful periods with large, black clots

Worse
Excessive emotions, including joy
Strong odors
Noise
Touch

Better
Lying down
Sleep

Food and Drink
Aversion to and worse from coffee
Aggravation from wine

Colchicum (Meadow saffron)

Key Symptoms
Morning sickness
Gout
Intolerance of odors, especially of food that is being cooked
Nausea and vomiting with nearly any complaint

Mind
Ultrasensitive to rudeness
Don't know what you want
Hard to please

Body
Highly sensitive to pain
Being touched feels like electric shocks in your body
Symptoms are worse from moving or turning your head
Bleeding and nausea at the same time

Breasts and Female Genitalia
Severe morning sickness with disgust at the sight, smell, or thought of food
Extreme restlessness during your last month of pregnancy
Thighs are cold after your period
Swelling of your vulva and clitoris

Worse
Motion
Loss of sleep

Better
Warmth
Rest

Food and Drink
Aggravation from eggs

Collinsonia (Stone-root)

Key Symptoms
Hemorrhoids
Digestive complaints during pregnancy
Hemorrhoids along with other problems

Mind
Ailments from emotional excitement
Indecision

Body
Feeling of sharp sticks or sand in your rectum
Hemorrhoids along with swelling of your face or lips
Varicose veins, constipation, and nausea with pregnancy
Hemorrhoids with heart palpitations

Breasts and Female Genitalia
Itching of vulva with hemorrhoids during pregnancy
Menstrual pain with hemorrhoids
Hemorrhoids with swelling of your labia and vagina
Prolapsed uterus with hemorrhoids

Worse
Hemorrhoids
Pregnancy
Night

Better
Warmth

Food and Drink
Desire for or aversion to cheese

Colocynthis (Bitter cucumber)

Key Symptoms
Abdominal cramping better from bending over
Illnesses after indignation or humiliation
Ailments from embarrassment

Mind
Easily offended
Indignant
Anger with your pain

Body
Violent, cramping abdominal pain
Diarrhea, nausea, and vomiting with the pain
Diarrhea from indignation

Breasts and Female Genitalia
Violent menstrual cramps that double you over
Clutching ovarian pain better from drawing legs up into abdomen
Menstrual pain is worse from eating or drinking
Ovarian pain better in knee-to-chest position

Worse
Becoming angry
Lying on the painless side

Better
Hard pressure

Food or Drink
Desire for bread and beer
Worse from potatoes and starchy food

Conium (Hemlock)

Key Symptoms
Benign and malignant tumors
Problems of glands, especially the breast
Stony, hard glands
Gradual paralysis

Mind
Sick after suppressing your sexual urges
Introversion
Blunted emotions
You don't want to be around anyone

Body
Breast tenderness or pain
Dizziness from turning the head or stooping
Fatigue, especially early in the morning before getting up

Breasts and Female Genitalia
Swollen and painful breasts before your periods
Engorgement of breasts and ovaries
Breasts are so painful that it hurts to move
Periods are irregular, late, and light

Worse
Sexual deprivation
Turning in bed

Better
Pressure
Stooping

Food and Drink
Worse from wine and milk
Desire for salt, sour foods, and coffee

Folliculinum (Estrone/follicular hormone)

Key Symptoms
Symptoms are worse from ovulation to menses
Conditions that begin after taking birth control pills
You feel you have lost your sense of self
Drained before your period

Mind
You feel dominated by others
Premenstrual depression
Mood swings before your period

Body
Ovulatory or premenstrual symptoms
All sorts of irregularities in your cycle
Premenstrual headaches
Premenstrual migraines

Breasts and Female Genitalia
Ovulatory problems such as spotting and ovarian cysts
Breasts swollen before period
Ovarian cysts and polycystic ovaries
Pain in ovaries during your period

Worse
From ovulation until your period
Heat
Touch and noise

Better
Fresh air

Food and Drink
Extreme food cravings before your period

Gelsemium (Yellow jasmine)

Key Symptoms
Fear of speaking in public
You're dizzy, drowsy, droopy, and dull when you have the flu
Wiped-out feeling
Ailments from fright

Mind
Everything seems like too much
Do not feel you can cope
You feel like giving up
Desire to be held so you don't shake

Body
You feel dull, heavy, and have no thirst
Loss of muscular power
Chills, weakness, and trembling
Menstrual pain with light flow and pain extending to back and hips

Breasts and Female Genitalia
Uterus feels heavy, sore, squeezed
Sleepy and exhausted during labor
Labor makes no progress even though os is fully dilated
Severe, sharp labor pains extending from uterus to back and hips

Worse
Fright
Shock
Surprise

Better
Shaking
Profuse urination

Food and Drink
Better from alcohol

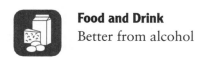

Hamamelis (Witch hazel)

Key symptoms
Hemorrhoids, varicose veins, and bleeding
Bruised, sore feeling, especially of the veins
Swelling and inflammation
Bleeding from injuries

Mind
You want others to respect you
You don't feel like studying or working
Irritability

Body
Varicose veins during pregnancy
Legs are so painful during pregnancy that you can't walk
Bleeding hemorrhoids
Nosebleed instead of your period

Breasts and Female Genitalia
Menstrual flow around ovulation only during the day
Dark, heavy periods with soreness of your abdomen
Painful hemorrhoids after a miscarriage
Your abdomen is sore following a miscarriage

Worse
Injuries or bruises
During the day
Pressure or touch

Better
Rest
Lying quietly

Food and Drink
Aversion to water

Ignatia (St. Ignatius bean)

Key Symptoms
Most common medicine immediately following grief or loss
Uncontrollable sobbing, loss of appetite, and extreme sadness
Great mood swings
Frequent sighing
Numbness and cramping anywhere in your body

Mind
High-strung and emotionally reactive
Upset after hurt or disappointment
Say or do the opposite of what others would expect

Body
Sensation of a lump in the throat, especially after grief
Symptoms that are just the opposite of what one would expect
Numbness and tingling
Pressure or tightness in your chest

Breasts and Female Genitalia
Miscarriage from grief or loss
Periods stop after grief
Menstrual cramping following loss or disappointment
Periods are irregular, early, too heavy or light

Worse
Grief or disappointment

IGNATIA
(St. Ignatius bean)

Better
Deep breathing
Changing positions

Food and Drink
Strong desire for or dislike of fruit
Desire for cheese

Kreosotum (Creosote)

Key Symptoms
Acrid, excoriating discharges
Irritability
Lots of problems around your period

Mind
Excited feeling premenstrually
Fear of sexual intimacy
Dreams and fear of sexual assault
You say you are well when you are very sick

Body
Throbbing all over the body
Burning pains as if on fire

Breasts and Female Genitalia
Vaginal discharge before and after your period
Burning vaginal discharge that irritates your labia
Severe headache before and during your period
Humming and buzzing sensations premenstrually

Worse
Pregnancy
Making love
Becoming chilled
After Period

Better
Warmth
Hot food

Food and Drink
Desire for meat

Lac caninum (Dog's milk)

Key symptoms
Symptoms alternate from side to side
Floating sensation
Difficulty with nurturing or being nurtured
Low self-esteem

Mind
You think others look down upon you
You feel like the underdog
Constant desire to wash your hands
Dreams of snakes

Body
Various throat problems
Breasts so painful that you must hold them going up and down the stairs
Sexual desire is easily aroused on touching genitals
Ravenous hunger

Breasts and Female Genitalia
Breasts painful and swollen before your period
Need to dry up breast milk

Loss of milk production while nursing
Period is hot, gushing, bright red, too early

Worse
Touch
Being jarred

Better
Open air

Food and Drink
Desire for pepper, mustard, and pungent foods

Lachesis (Bushmaster snake)

Key Symptoms
Symptoms are worse on the left side of the body
Symptoms that move from left to right
Symptoms that are worse on waking or after sleep
Fear of snakes

Mind
You are quite intense
You are a talker
Jump from one subject to the next
Jealous and suspicious

Body
You can't stand tight clothing around your neck
Purplish varicose veins or skin eruptions

Breasts and Female Genitalia
Hot flashes
Premenstrual syndrome rage
Left-sided premenstrual headaches
Left ovarian pain

Worse
After sleep
Slightest touch
Suppression of emotions or symptoms

Better
Discharges of any kind
Onset of your period
Expressing your emotions

Food or Drink
Desire for starchy food and oysters

Lactuca virosa (Wild lettuce)

Key Symptoms
Sense of lightness of body as if swimming
Tightness of whole body, especially chest
Faulty milk production

Mind
Restlessness with fear and anxiety
Can't remember what you wanted to say
Disturbed sleep due to anxiety

Body
Chest tightness as if you are about to suffocate
Sleepiness while having a bowel movement

Cannot lie on your back
Urine smells like violets

Breasts and Female Genitalia
No breast milk
Painful vaginal discharge
Periods are too early and too frequent

Worse
Touch
Pressure
Warm room

Better
Outdoor exercise

Food and Drink
Desire for milk
Feel worse from drinking milk

Lilium tigrinum (Tiger lily)

Key Symptoms
Very high sexual energy
Problems of the uterus and ovaries
Must keep busy
Hurried

Mind
Strong religious interest combined with strong sex drive
Wild feeling
Premenstrual irritability
You want to do several things at the same time

Body
Throbbing feeling all over your body
Intense vaginal itching before period
Burning in your palms and soles
Cutting pain in your abdomen premenstrually

Breasts and Female Genitalia
Dragging feeling in pelvis as if your organs will fall out
Premenstrual breast tenderness
Neuralgic pains in uterus worse from the pressure of clothing
Periods are early, light, dark, clotted, and smell strong

Worse
Night
Menses

Better
Urinating
Eating

Food and Drink
Desire for meat
Aversion to food in general

Lycopodium (Club moss)

Key Symptoms
Symptoms that are right-sided or move from right to left
Desire for warm or room-temperature drinks
Worse from 4 to 8 P.M.
Stage fright

Mind
Issues of self-confidence
You appear confident but are really afraid

Fear of taking on new things
Irritability in the morning on waking

Body
Gas and bloating
Bloating after eating even a small amount of food
You don't like tight-fitting clothes around your abdomen
Difficulty gaining weight

Breasts and Female Genitalia
Right ovarian cysts or pain
Dry, burning vaginal pain worse from making love
Periods are suppressed for months at a time
Breast milk without being pregnant

Worse
Pressure of clothing, especially around abdomen
Eating

Better
Warm drinks

Food and Drink
Strong desire for sweets

Magnesia phosphorica (Magnesium phosphate)

Key Symptoms
Cramping pains in the abdomen
Pain relieved from warm applications and pressure
Feel groggy in the morning on waking
Insomnia due to indigestion

Mind
Feeling of not being nurtured
You talk a lot about your problems
Silent and moody
Disgruntled

Body
Right-sided problems
Intense, sore, bruised feeling in the abdomen
Abdominal bloating with a desire to loosen the clothes around the abdomen
Liver problems

Breasts and Female Genitalia
Menstrual cramps relieved by bending double, warmth, and pressure
Pain is much better once your period begins
Menstrual flow is dark and too early
Swelling of the labia
Ovarian pain

Worse
Cold
Night
Exhaustion

Better
Hot bath
Doubling over
Pressure

Food and Drink
Aggravation from milk

Mercurius corrosivus (Mercuric chloride)

Key Symptoms
Tremendous urge to urinate
Urinating does not relieve the urge
Spasm of bladder and rectum

Mind
Anxious and restless
Difficulty thinking and speaking clearly
You don't understand what others say to you

Body
Intense burning in the urethra
Urine is hot and burning
Urine is passed a drop at a time with great pain
Blood in urine

Breasts and Female Genitalia
Nipples swell, crack, and bleed
Period is too heavy and comes too early
Cervical erosion
Acrid vaginal discharge

Worse
After urinating
After a bowel movement

Better
Rest

Food and Drink
Desire for cold food
Unquenchable thirst

Natrum muriaticum (Sodium chloride)

Key Symptoms
You are vulnerable to having your feelings hurt
You put up a wall so you won't get hurt
Want to be left alone when you're not feeling well
Don't want to cry in front of others

Mind

History of grief or disappointment in relationships
Overly sensitive to the slightest reprimand or insult
If your feelings get hurt, you withdraw
Deeply affected by music

Body

Headaches from exposure to the heat or sun
Canker sores in the mouth
Cold sores on the lips
Crack in the center of the lower lip

Breasts and Female Genitalia

Dryness of the vagina
Aversion to making love
Thick, white vaginal discharge
Burning in the vagina during sex

Worse

10 A.M.
Exposure to the sun

Better

Open air

Food and Drink

Desire for salty food, pasta, bread, lemons
Aversion to slimy food

Nux vomica (Quaker's button)

Key Symptoms

Muscle tension, cramping, and spasms
Hard-driving and demanding of yourself and others
Craving for stimulants
Chilly

Mind

Excessive concern about business
Want to be the first and the best
Quite impatient
Easily offended

Body

Waking at 3:00 to 4:00 A.M. with your mind full of ideas
Heartburn that is worse from spicy foods
Constipation without a desire to have a bowel movement
Heightened sensitivity to light, noise, sound, and other stimuli

Breasts and Female Genitalia

Menstrual cramps extending to the whole body
Fainting with labor pains
Profuse, yellow vaginal discharge premenstrually that stains your pants
Periods come too early

Worse

Abuse of alcohol or drugs
Eating too much food or excessively spicy food
Cold

Better

Discharges from the body
Rest

Food and Drink

Desire spicy or fatty foods, coffee, alcohol, and tobacco

Petroleum (Coal oil)

Key Symptoms

Motion sickness
Severely dry skin to the point of cracking and bleeding

Mind
Easily lost and confused
Get lost in familiar places
Difficulty making a decision
Quarrelsome

Body
Ragged, chapped, cracked fingertips and heels
Heartburn
Must get up at night to eat

Breasts and Female Genitalia
Genital herpes
Aversion to sex
Itching with the menstrual flow
Soreness and wetness of labia, with violent itching

Worse
Travel
Cold weather

Better
Dry weather
Warm air

Food and Drink
Desire for beer
Averse to meat, fats, and cooked or hot foods

Phellandrium (Water dropwort)

Key Symptoms
Mastitis
Unbearable breast pain between nursing
Right-sided symptoms
Bronchitis

Mind

You feel anxious about your health

It feels as if someone is behind you

Peeved

Meditative

Body

Menstrual cramps not alleviated by sitting, standing, or lying down

Heavy menstrual flow only in the morning or evening

Overpowering sleepiness during work

Breasts and Female Genitalia

Pain in the right breast extending to the back between the shoulder blades

Breast pain during your period

Breast pain extends to the back or abdomen

Worse

Cold air

Better

While nursing

Food and Drink

Everything tastes sweet

Craving for acidic foods and cold milk

Phosphorus

Key Symptoms

Bleeding and bruising

Extroverted

Great thirst for cold drinks

Respiratory problems

Mind

Lively, friendly, sociable person
You always want company
Very caring about others
Tendency to be worried and fearful

Body

Woozy and disoriented days after anesthesia
Waking during night with hunger
Hypoglycemia
Symptoms are worse from lying on your left side

Breasts and Female Genitalia

Excessive, bright-red menstrual bleeding without clots
Periods last too long
Genital warts that bleed easily
Gushing between your periods from fibroids or cysts

Worse

Spicy foods
Warm foods
Fasting

Better

Lying on the right side
Being around other people
Eating

Food and Drink

Desire for salty and spicy food, chocolate, chicken
Desire for carbonated drinks

Phytolacca (Poke-root)

Key Symptoms

Glandular swelling and inflammation, especially breast, tonsils, and parotid glands (mumps)

Right-sided symptoms
Mastitis

Mind
Want to die during mastitis
Indifference and apathy
Lack of embarrassment

Body
Soreness all over your body
Enlarged lymph nodes in your armpit
Glandular swellings with heat and inflammation
Restlessness

Breasts and Female Genitalia
Breast is heavy, swollen, tender, and stone-hard
Hard nodules in your breast
Discharge from your nipple long after weaning
Breast pain during nursing that spreads all through your body

Worse
Night
Cold, damp weather

Better
Lying on your stomach
Supporting your breasts

Food or Drink
Ravenous appetite soon after eating

Pulsatilla (Windflower)

Key Symptoms
Puberty, menstrual problems, pregnancy, menopause
Moods and symptoms change very quickly

You cry very easily
Prefer to be outside in the open air

Mind
Soft, affectionate, motherly
Desire for attention and company
Indecisive
Highly emotional

Body
Thick, bland, yellowish-green discharges
Ailments from suppressing any bodily discharge
Dry mouth but no thirst
Easily overheated and uncomfortable in warm, stuffy rooms

Breasts and Female Genitalia
Thick, milky, or creamy vaginal discharge
Absence of periods
Irregular, clotted, changeable menstrual periods
Swelling of breasts after weaning

Worse
Heat
Rich foods

Better
Open air
Cold applications, food, or drink

Food and Drink
Desire for fats, rich foods, peanut butter
Aggravation from meat and rich foods

Sabina (Savine)

Key Symptoms
Problems of female pelvic organs
Miscarriage

Women's problems after miscarriage
Uterine bleeding with bright-red blood and dark clots

Mind
Highly irritable and anxious
Extreme sensitivity to music
Sensitive to noise

Body
Tendency to bleed
Feeling of fullness and swelling in the blood vessels
Hot-blooded with inflamed joints
Heel problems

Breasts and Female Genitalia
Threatened miscarriage, especially in the third month
Drawing pain in the small of the back, penetrating right through the pelvis to the pubis
Blood is bright red, thin, and liquid or has dark-red clots
Blood comes out in gushes and is more profuse on movement

Worse
Heat
Music is intolerable
Night

Better
Cold

Food and Drink
Crave sour, juicy, refreshing things

Sanguinaria (Blood-root)

Key Symptoms
Congestion of blood to the head, chest, abdomen
Right-sided remedy

Burning and throbbing
Warm-blooded, especially around menopause

Mind
Grumbly
You make mountains out of mole hills
Inertia
Feeling of dread

Body
Red cheeks
Burning pain in palms and soles of feet
Right shoulder pain
Dry mucous membranes

Breasts and Female Genitalia
Hot flashes
Burning vaginal discharge
Breasts sore and enlarged at menopause
Bright-red, clotted bleeding between periods around menopause

Worse
Menopause
Sun

Better
Lying on your back

Food and Drink
Craving for spicy and pungent food

Sarsaparilla (Wild licorice)

Key Symptoms
One of the best medicines for bladder infections in women
Burning at the urethra at the close of urination
Right-sided symptoms

Mind

Easily offended

Depression and anxiety from the pain

Sad for no apparent reason

Body

Severe, almost unbearable pain at the close of urination

Constant desire to urinate but little or nothing comes out

You may only be able to urinate while standing

Violent urge to urinate with stubborn constipation

Breasts and Female Genitalia

Menstrual cramps with extreme pain in lower abdomen and back

Cramps extend down thighs

Fainting, sweating, vomiting, and diarrhea with cramps

Breast soreness with menstrual cramps

Worse

At the close of urination

Getting cold and wet

Better

Standing

Food or Drink

Bread disagrees

Drinking water causes vomiting

Sepia (Cuttlefish ink)

Key Symptoms

Hormonal problems in women

Lack of sexual desire

Desire for vigorous exercise or dancing
Desire for vinegar, pickles, and other sour foods

Mind
Grumpy, weepy
Indifference or aversion to your family
Feel stuck, unmotivated, trapped
You would rather be left alone

Body
Morning sickness
Constipation
Loss of urine from coughing or sneezing
Never well since pregnancy, miscarriage, or taking birth control pills

Breasts and Female Genitalia
Yellowish-green or white, foul-smelling vaginal discharge
Lots of vaginal itching
You feel as if your pelvic organs will fall out
Shriveled breasts

Worse
Pregnancy, miscarriage, abortion
4:00 to 6:00 P.M.
Cold air

Better
Vigorous exercise
Dancing

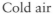

Food and Drink
Craving for vinegar and pickles
Desire for chocolate

Silica (Flint)

Key Symptoms
Low stamina and energy
Obstinate constipation
Abscesses
Swollen glands

Mind
Must meet the standards of others
Shy in social situations and appearing in public
Proper, polite, refined
Particular about how things should be

Body
Abscesses, cysts, or boils anywhere in the body
Bad-smelling or sour perspiration, especially from your feet
Problems with your nails or teeth
Swollen glands, often filled with pus

Breasts and Female Genitalia
Milky, burning, profuse, gushing vaginal discharge
Milk suppressed or absent
Thin, bad-tasting milk that baby refuses
Sensitivity and itching of vulva and vagina

Worse
Cold draft
Suppressed perspiration

Better
Wrapping up

Food and Drink
Worse from cold food and fats
Desire for eggs

Staphysagria (Stavesacre)

Key Symptoms
Bladder infections after sex
Symptoms from suppressed anger
Ailments after insult, humiliation, or rudeness
Toothaches, headaches

Mind
Mild and gentle
You tend to give in
Self-blame
Trembling from anger

Body
Bladder infection after too much sex or sex with a new partner
Frequent urge to urinate, but nothing comes out
Bladder does not feel empty, even right after urinating
Burning in urethra during urination, or especially when not urinating

Breasts and Female Genitalia
Absence of periods after indignation
High sexual energy and tendency to masturbate
Painful sensitivity of the vagina and labia on sitting down
Ovarian pain extending to the thighs

Worse
Sexual intercourse

Better
Warmth

Food and Drink
Desire for or aversion to milk
Craving for sweets and tobacco

Sulphur

Key Symptoms
Hot-blooded
Skin eruptions with lots of itching
Burning pains anywhere in the body
Left-sided symptoms

Mind
Opinionated and critical
Busy mind with daydreaming
Philosophical, creative, imaginative
Disorganized

Body
Feet become unbearably hot; must uncover them
Diarrhea with sudden urging
Bad-smelling sweat and discharges
Heartburn

Breasts and Female Genitalia
Hot flashes worse at night in bed
Hotter after a hot bath or shower
Offensive odor of the vaginal area
Itching and soreness in vulva and vagina

Worse
Heat
11:00 A.M.
After taking a hot bath or shower

Better
Cooling off
Sweating

Food and Drink
Desire for sweets; spicy, fatty foods; alcohol
Aversion to eggs

Tabacum (Tobacco)

Key Symptoms

Deathly nauseous with violent vomiting, worse from any motion

Symptoms such as nausea and dizziness come in waves

Motion sickness

Your face looks deathly pale

Mind

Wretched feeling

Sudden anxiety

Discouraged, resigned

Anxiety is better from crying

Body

Incapacitating nausea

Severe vomiting with lots of spitting

Nausea better from uncovering the abdomen

Nausea worse from opening the eyes

Breasts and Female Genitalia

Morning sickness

Nausea during period or menopause

Severe itching of entire body during pregnancy

Worse

Traveling in a car or on a boat

Opening your eyes

Better

Fresh air

Cold applications

Uncovering your abdomen

Food and Drink

Desire for tobacco

Veratrum album (White hellebore)

Key Symptoms
Severe abdominal cramping
Chilliness and cold sweat
Collapse with blueness of skin
Desire for icy, cold food and drinks

Mind
Mental overstimulation
Always busy
Concern about your social status
Think you know best

Body
Abdominal cramping with chills, vomiting, diarrhea, and cold sweats
Symptoms are worse before your period
Profuse vomiting, purging, salivation, perspiration, urination
Simultaneous vomiting and diarrhea

Breasts and Female Genitalia
Violent menstrual cramps with diarrhea, chills, vomiting
Fainting with menstrual pain at the least movement
Very high sexual desire before your period
Miscarriage with cold sweat, vomiting, and thirst for cold water

Worse
Cold drinks
Exertion

Better
Warmth
Warm drinks
Walking around

Food or Drink
Crave ice, cold drinks, juicy fruit, salty foods

PART FIVE

Enhancing Your Healing

CHAPTER 15

Complements to Homeopathic Healing
Essential Elements of a Balanced Lifestyle

The following twenty-five tips came to me spontaneously as I wrote an article ten years ago, and patients still tell me they are quite helpful. I hope that they will benefit you as well.

1. *Be present. Live each moment to the fullest.* Few of us focus our total attention on the here and now. We are trapped by the pain of the past and fear of the future and by forever looking to fulfill another desire. If you concentrate on what is happening right now, your experience of life will be infinitely richer and you'll actually be there to enjoy it. I recently attended an evening presentation by Ekhardt Tolle, author of *The Power of Now.* He shared something that I will not forget. "I never hope to experience another moment any more complete and perfect than this one."

2. *Let love be your highest priority.* Love yourself, those dear to you, family, friends, colleagues, neighbors, and your cohabitants of this planet in all their forms. When all is said and done and your time on this earth is over, the only thing that will matter is how much you were able to love.

3. *Surround yourself with people who bring out the best in you.* Most of us have been on the receiving end of more than enough negative messages. Choose to give and receive love and friendship from people who encourage your creativity and fulfillment of your life's dreams and are supportive in good times as well as bad. Be open to constructive criticism, but screen out inappropriate criticism and negativity.

4. *There is no limit to the extent you can help and serve others.* Nothing cures a depression more quickly than going to the pediatric ward of a hospital or serving Thanksgiving dinner to the homeless. Being of use to others reminds you how much

you have to give and how much better off you are than many other people. While finishing this project I had the opportunity to participate in a one-day-a-year service event in our small community. This being my first year, imagine my surprise at finding four hundred of my neighbors gathered to work on thirty-two homes in need of good, hard work. In one day, $200,000 worth of labor and $400,000 worth of materials were lovingly and humbly donated. It was one of the most inspiring days I've ever spent.

5. *Heal your relationship with your family.* It is no accident that you ended up with the parents you did, although it may seem that way in your most difficult moments. They can be your greatest teachers or your most formidable adversaries. Being around your family is likely to trigger any of your unresolved issues. Face them and, if possible, forgive, heal, and move on, whether or not your family is still alive. The same is true with siblings.

6. *Take care of unfinished business.* It is never too late to heal your anger, resentment, fears, worries, insecurities, and any other emotions or concerns that stand in the way of your happiness. Whether it is through mediation, psychotherapy, meditation, prayer, or any other method, clear the air as soon as you possibly can. You haven't a clue as to what the future will bring.

I would like to share a very poignant story from one of my favorite books, *Small Miracles of Love and Friendship.*[1] Tracy's father had been gruff and unexpressive for as long as she could remember. His inability to demonstrate his love for her became so painful to Tracy that she withdrew her own warmth and affection from him so that it would not be rebuffed. One evening when he was up in years, Tracy and her mother somehow coaxed him to go out on the town and, even more amazingly, he agreed to dance with his daughter for the very first time in her life. He was finally able to confide his regret at being remiss about his duties as a father. Struck by his inability to maintain eye contact during their dance, Tracy finally whispered, tears in her eyes, "Why is it so hard for you to *look* at me?" Her father's misty-eyed response: "Because I love you so much."

At that point Tracy, left speechless by his touching answer, excused herself to the restroom. When she came back, she was met with screams and commotion. Her father, ashen gray and slumped over in his chair, had succumbed to a heart attack. The precious dance that they shared was their first and last.

7. *Forgive yourself first, then others.* On some level, however misguided, we are all trying to do the best we can at each and every moment, even though it may not show. You will suffer much more, in one form or another, by continuing to harbor resentment, maybe even through a physical illness. It only takes one to forgive. If the other person is willing, that's even better, but this is often not the case.

8. *Be compassionate.* It feels wonderful to express kindness and caring to others. Just a smile or a kind word can make someone's day. We get so self-absorbed and busy in our lives that it is easy to forget the little things that make such a difference. Step back and show others the special caring that each of us deserves.

9. *Take good care of your body. It's yours for life.* If you treat your body with respect and care, it can be your friend for life. Listen to your body and respond to its requests before they turn into urgent demands. Know when to push the envelope and when to give it a rest. If you're not feeling up to par, change your plans and take time to heal.

10. *Discover the foods that work best for you and eat them most of the time.* Your body will usually tell you what it needs unless your desires are overpowering. There are many diets and eating plans. Find one that helps you feel good and maintain a healthful weight. Eat natural and organic foods, keep sugar at a minimum, and limit caffeine and alcohol.

11. *Supplement a healthful diet with high-quality vitamins and minerals.* You don't need to fill a medicine chest with supplements in order to remain vital and healthy, but you won't get all of your nutritional needs met through food alone. Our environment just isn't as pure as we'd like, and junk foods deplete nutrients. Consider nutritional supplements as part of your investment in a long and healthful life.

12. *Find an exercise program that you enjoy and stick with it.* Get aerobic for at least twenty minutes three or four times a week. If you are perimenopausal, make working out part of your ongoing fitness program. Whether it be tennis, swimming, running, yoga, dancing, racquetball, walking, kayaking, martial arts, or whatever, choose sports or activities you really like and that are realistic for your lifestyle. If you tire of one, switch to another. Just do it!

13. *Keep it simple!* Living in a world of beepers, cell phones, laptops, e-mail, and sound bytes has created far more complexity than ever before. It can take a concerted effort to keep your life manageable, but it's worth it. With every additional complication comes attachment and responsibility until you don't have time for the things that really matter.

14. *Invite the child in you to come out and play.* Make time for fun and relaxation. Fly a kite, blow a bubble, take a kid to the zoo, purr with your kitty. Reenact what you most loved when you were growing up or what you would have liked to have done but never did.

15. *Don't take yourself and your life too seriously.* Life isn't nearly as important as we make it out to be. You can make your day-to-day events into a matter of life and death if they don't unfold according to plan. Worry causes ulcers and lots of other problems and usually doesn't change a thing, so why bother?

16. *Ask for help when you need it.* You can't possibly handle and fix every problem that arises yourself. You need help. And it warms others' hearts to be able to help you out when you're in need. Help is available and can come from the most unexpected places. Just don't forget to ask for it.

17. *Keep breathing!* There is no better way to calm and de-stress yourself than to concentrate on your breath. Slow and deep, nice and easy, in and out. It's very hard to worry about anything as long as you're thinking about breathing. Then life becomes one inhalation and exhalation after another and all is well. The ancient yogis used to measure lifetimes in terms of the number of breaths rather than in years. The longer each breath, the longer your life.

18. *Cultivate peace of mind and don't let anything get in its way.* Nothing is more essential than feeling at peace with yourself, and having a deep, abiding sense of quiet and contentment. Find a place of refuge, inner or outer, where you can access that peace whenever you desire until it occupies more and more of your life.

19. *Take responsibility for your life and your actions.* Be honest with yourself about what you need to own up to and to change. Denial is no fun for you or those around you. If you make a mistake, admit it, realize that we all make mistakes, and move forward. Make amends for what you need to, switch courses or opinions if they don't serve you, and admit to yourself what parts of you need work and plan a course of action.

20. *Patience is not only a virtue but rather a necessity.* Not only does racing around distract us and rob us of our spontaneity, but it causes ulcers! Many years ago a friend of mine who teaches yoga, taught me a very effective mantra, "Nowhere to go. Nothing to do." Some of the wisest beings of all time have learned to simply be still. It is being, not doing, that brings happiness.

21. *Let nature be your companion.* The preciousness of a gorgeous sunset, the magic of snow glistening on a distant mountain, the power of roaring waves against a rocky cliff—they take your breath away and, somehow, make the world stop. We live on a phenomenally beautiful planet. Every rose, eagle, starfish, and starry night is a gift.

22. *Give yourself to intimacy.* Touching, caressing, and making love are profound ways to connect with another human being in an atmosphere of tenderness and sacredness. Whether you are heterosexual or lesbian, are in a committed relationship or not, are able to have children or not, have suffered sexual abuse, or have physical impairments that limit your enjoyment of sex, intimacy is an expression of our life force and can be appreciated in many different ways.

23. *Treat Mother Earth lovingly. You can't live without her.* We live in an era of endangered species and endangered indigenous peoples. Overpopulation, overcrowding, overuse of the Earth's resources, and greed are changing the face of our planet. If

you do not make a personal commitment to saving the planet, she may not be around, at least in her current bounty, for the generations to come.

24. ***Connect with your Creator on a regular basis.*** Pray, meditate, and contemplate daily so that you can remain connected with God, Consciousness, Spirit, Higher Self, or whatever you call that universal oneness. It is this deep connection that will bring you the greatest happiness of your life.

25. ***Do what you love. Health and healing will follow.*** You have your own unique talents and life purpose. The more you learn about your gifts and open yourself to the lessons you are here to learn, the easier it will be to find work you love. If you are passionate about your livelihood, you are much more likely to be in love with life, which is one of the most essential components of health.

CHAPTER 16

The Promise of Healing the Whole You

What If You Were Completely Healed?

A VISION OF HEALING FOR YOURSELF

What exactly does healing mean to you? If you happen to be confined to a wheelchair, as a result of a head or spinal injury, such as Christopher Reeve, healing may be the ability to one day walk on your own and to breathe without the assistance of a machine. If you have suffered a number of miscarriages, your pinnacle of healing might be to have a healthy child. Or you may long to be free of excruciating menstrual pain, maddening PMS, or the fibroid that weighs on you, literally and figuratively. If you suffer from depression, anxiety, or obsessive-compulsive disorder, healing may be the opportunity to wake up morning after morning in good spirits and free of worry. For many of us, healing means to live a vibrant, happy, and long life surrounded by loved ones. Or to save the planet. In the case of spiritual aspirants, healing might take the form of becoming enlightened or ensuring that all others are able to do so. Healing is quite relative.

What would healing look like for *you*? Put aside everything else for a few minutes, close your eyes, let go, and allow yourself to experience a state of deep and abiding peacefulness. Relax. Breathe. Now ask yourself what it would look like for you to be healed on all levels. Once you let go of concepts, don't be surprised if total healing looks different than you thought it might. Imagine, visualize, or contemplate what your life would be like, what would be different, and how your life would unfold if you were absolutely healed. Your relationship with yourself and others, your body, career, spiritual life, lifestyle, day-to-day experiences. Now take a moment to assess any and all obstacles to your being totally healed, whatever that means to you. For each obstacle, ask yourself what needs to happen in order to remove the obstruction. Then, once again, hold in your mind that image of yourself being fully healed. Think of all the ways you could contribute to and serve others so that they, too, could be healed. Start and end each day with this thought and observe how your life evolves.

HOMEOPATHY CAN HELP REMOVE LIMITATIONS TO FREEDOM

Homeopathy is a form of energy medicine that has the potential to bring your life into balance. An important aspect of mental healing is clarity of thinking and the elimination of confusion. From that place of clarity, you can more readily envision how you fit into the world and accept more gracefully what comes your way. Homeopathy can enhance that process by removing any limitations to mental freedom, as well as your physical and emotional blocks.

One of the greatest joys of being a homeopath is to watch my patients develop that clarity of mind, acceptance, and vision regardless of, and sometimes as a by-product of, the pain and suffering that they may have experienced in their lives.

Meg, mentioned earlier in the context of healing after sexual abuse, describes this process, as it developed for her, far better than I could:

Meg's Dream

"My teenage years were tremendously hard for me, especially dealing with my parents. During this time, I was quite influenced by the human rights movements that were taking shape in society around me. I particularly recall, at that time, identifying with Martin Luther King Jr.'s 'I Have a Dream' speech. As his message of freedom and equality was being disseminated from the podium to his supporters, then broadcast throughout the United States into the suburbs, and finally into the home where I sat watching it on TV with my parents, something very powerful happened to me. I began to recognize that I, like many of his supporters and those in his congregation, was nodding my agreement of his truth and that I, too, had a dream. A dream that was very, very different from anything I'd ever been exposed to before. I've found that a very intrinsic part of the healing process for me has been the ability to carry somewhere inside myself some kind of a vision of what being healthy is really all about for myself. This vision is available to me, no matter how obscured my mind may be temporarily, and, throughout the course of my healing process, I have become able to allow myself to progressively and steadily connect with that vision."

The most profound benefits of homeopathy often occur over time. Dramatic improvements in symptoms and overall health can occur within weeks or months of taking a medicine. But each of us still live with our state: the fundamental, and frequently mistaken, beliefs and perceptions that guide and often limit us in our lives. Over time, with effective homeopathic treatment, our states can become less limiting and we become freer to be ourselves. Meg is a changed woman compared to the timid, unhappy, self-conscious, self-deprecatory person I met nine years ago. Homeopathy, of course, is not completely responsible for her transformation, and she still has plenty of room to learn and grow, but she is the first to admit that it has helped her tremendously.

Homeopathy has the potential, or promise, to catalyze a healing process that reaches much further than you can imagine. It has the potential to remove your obstacles, to cure so that you can be all that you are meant to be.

A CHAIN REACTION OF HEALING

Once you are happier and healthier, your joy and well-being will be contagious. I was quite moved by an article that I read in the Seattle newspaper. "Every so often, something happens that restores one's faith in the milk—or make that the latté—of random human kindness. Take the recent incident at Romeo's Drive-Thru Espresso." A woman driver, who happened to be a regular customer satisfying her urge for a morning fix in latté land, pulled up to the stand just before dawn on a cold morning in late December. After having ordered a white chocolate mocha to warm herself up, in a holiday spirit, she also paid for a drink for the stranger in the car behind her. Stunned by her generosity, he decided he'd better do the same. And so it went, continuously, as nearly one hundred drivers passed through, from 6:45 A.M. until the stand closed at 2:00 P.M. And what did the last motorist do? He handed the espresso manager a five-dollar bill and instructed her to buy coffee the following morning for the woman who started the chain.[1] Who knows, maybe it still hasn't ended!

And so it is, when we are healed. That freedom allows us, in turn, to spread the healing far and wide. Whether it be the more than half of the world's population that goes to sleep hungry, our beleaguered planet with its growing number of endangered species, or the many of us who suffer on so many levels, may we all be part of an unbroken chain of love and compassion that allows us all to be healed.

Appendix: Expanding Your Knowledge of Homeopathy

RECOMMENDED READING

Natural Healing for Women

Arnot, Bob. *The Breast Cancer Prevention Diet.* Boston: Little, Brown and Company, 1999.

Austin, Steve, and Cathy Hitchcock. *Breast Cancer: What You Should Know (but May Not Be Told) About Prevention, Diagnosis, and Treatment.* Roseville, CA: Prima Publishing, 1994.

Duncker, Patricia and Vicky Wilson. *Cancer Through the Eyes of Ten Women.* San Francisco, CA: HarperCollins Publishers, 1996.

Ford, Gillian. *Listening to Your Hormones: From PMS to Menopause, Every Woman's Complete Guide.* Roseville, CA: Prima Publishing, 1997.

Fore, Robert, and Rorie Fore. *Survivors Guide to Breast Cancer: A Couple's Story of Faith, Hope, and Love.* Macon, GA: Peake Road, 1998.

Heynen, Jim. *One Hundred Over 100: Moments with One Hundred North American Centenarians.* Golden, CO: Fulcrum Publishing, 1990.

Hudson, Tori. *Women's Encyclopedia of Natural Medicine: Alternative Therapies and Integrative Medicine.* Lincolnwood, IL: Keats, 1999.

Joseph, Barbara. *My Healing from Breast Cancer: A Physician's Personal Story of Recovery and Transformation.* New Canaan, CT: Keat Publishing, Inc., 1996.

Kahane, Deborah Hobler. *No Less a Woman: Femininity, Sexuality and Breast Cancer.* Alameda, CA: Hunter House, Inc., 1990.

Kitchener Cone, Faye. *Making Sense of Menopause.* New York: Simon and Schuster, 1993.

Lark, Susan. *The Estrogen Decision Self Help Book.* Berkeley, CA: Celestial Arts, 1995.

Lark, Susan. *Fibroid Tumors and Endometriosis Self Help Book.* Berkeley, CA: Celestial Arts, 1993.

Lark, Susan. *The Lark Letter.* A monthly newsletter covering women's health and healing issues. (1-877-4DRLARK for information and to subscribe.)

Lark, Susan. *The Menopause Self Help Book.* Berkeley, CA: Celestial Arts, 1992.

Lark, Susan. *Menstrual Cramps Self Help Book.* Berkeley, CA: Celestial Arts, 1995.

Lark, Susan. *PMS Self Help Book.* Berkeley, CA: Celestial Arts, 1984.

LaTour, Kathy. *The Breast Cancer Companion.* New York: Avon Books, 1993.

Lee, John. *What Your Doctor May Not Tell You About Menopause: The Breakthrough Book on Natural Progesterone.* New York: Warner Books, 1996.

Love, Susan. *Dr. Susan Love's Breast Book.* New York: Addison-Wesley, 1995.

Love, Susan. *Dr. Susan Love's Hormone Book: Making Informed Choices About Menopause.* New York: Times Books, 1998.

Murray, Michael, and Joseph Pizzorno. *Encyclopedia of Natural Medicine, Revised 2nd Edition.* Roseville, CA: Prima Publishing, 1997.

Northrup, Christiane. *Women's Bodies, Women's Wisdom.* New York: Bantam Books, 1998.

Ojeda, Linda. *Menopause Without Medicine.* Alameda, CA: Hunter House Inc. Publishers, 1992.

Sheehy, Gail. *The Silent Passage: Menopause.* New York: Random House, 1992.

Weed, Susun. *Breast Cancer? Breast Health! The Wise Woman Way.* Woodstock, New York: Ash Tree Publishing, 1996.

Weed, Susun. *Menopausal Years the Wise Woman Way: Alternative Approaches for Women 30–90.* Woodstock, NY: Ash Tree Publishing, 1992.

Homeopathy

Bellavite, Paolo, and Andrea Signorini. *Homeopathy: A Frontier in Medical Science.* Berkeley, CA: North Atlantic, 1995.

Castro, Miranda. *Homeopathy for Pregnancy, Birth, and Your Baby's First Year.* New York: St. Martins Press, 1993.

Idarius, Betty. *The Homeopathic Childbirth Manual.* Ukiah, CA: Idarius Press, 1996.

Ikenze, Ifeoma. *Menopause and Homeopathy: A Guide for Women in Midlife.* Berkeley, CA: North Atlantic Books, 1998.

Lockie, Andrew and Nicola Geddes. *The Women's Guide to Homeopathy.* New York: St. Martins Press, 1994.

Moskowitz, Richard. *Homeopathic Medicines for Pregnancy and Childbirth.* Berkeley, CA: North Atlantic Press, 1992.

Perko, Sandra. *Homeopathy for the Modern, Pregnant Woman and Her Infant.* San Antonio, TX: Benchmark Homeopathic Publications, 1997.

Reichenberg-Ullman, Judyth, and Robert Ullman. *Prozac-Free: Homeopathic Medicine for Depression, Anxiety and Other Mental and Emotional Problems*. Roseville, CA: Prima Publishing, 1996.

Reichenberg-Ullman, Judyth, and Robert Ullman. *Rage-Free Kids: Homeopathic Medicine for Defiant, Aggressive, and Violent Children*. Roseville, CA: Prima Publishing, 1999.

Reichenberg-Ullman, Judyth, and Robert Ullman. *Ritalin-Free Kids: Safe and Effective Homeopathic Medicine for ADD and Other Behavioral and Learning Problems*. Roseville, CA: Prima Publishing, 1996.

Ullman, Robert and Judyth Reichenberg-Ullman. *Homeopathic Self-Care: The Quick and Easy Guide for the Whole Family*. Roseville, CA: 1997.

Ullman, Robert, and Judyth Reichenberg-Ullman. *The Patient's Guide to Homeopathic Medicine*. Edmonds, WA: Picnic Point Press, 1995.

Homeopathic Book Distributors

Picnic Point Press
131 3rd Avenue, North
Edmonds, WA 98020
Phone: (800) 398-1151
Fax: (425) 670-0319
Web site: www.healthyhomeopathy.com
Carries our books and kits only.

Homeopathic Educational Services
2124 Kittredge Street
Berkeley, CA 94704
Phone: (510) 649-0294 (for inquiries or catalogs);
   (800) 359-9051 (orders only)

The Minimum Price
250 H Street
P.O. Box 2187
Blaine, WA 98231
Phone: (800) 663-8272

Referral Sources for Homeopathic Practitioners

Homeopathic practitioners vary widely regarding their level of medical or psychiatric training and experience, licensing or certification, expertise, and style of practice. Not all of the practitioners in the following directories necessarily use the same methods I have described in this book or are qualified to treat patients with serious mental illness.

Homeopathic Academy of Naturopathic Physicians (HANP)
12132 S.E. Foster Place
Portland, OR 97266
Phone: (503) 761-3298
Fax: (503) 762-1929

The National Center for Homeopathy (NCH)
801 N. Fairfax, #306
Alexandria, VA 22314
Phone: (703) 548-7790
Fax: (703) 548-7792

Council for Homeopathic Certification (CHC)
1709 Seabright Avenue
Santa Cruz, CA 95062
Phone: (408) 421-0565

American Institute of Homeopathy (AIH)
10418 Whithead Street
Fairfax, VA 22030
Phone: (703) 246-9501

North American Society of Homeopaths (NASH)
1122 East Pike Street, Suite 1122
Seattle, WA 98122
Phone: (206) 720-7000

How You Can Help

Homeopathy Without Borders
Nancy Kelly
P.O. Box 570
Bolinas, CA 94924
Phone: (415) 868-2950

Our mission is to provide humanitarian aid, homeopathic education, and treatment, while serving as partners with communities in need. Donations accepted.

Notes

CHAPTER 1

1. Tizon, Alex. "Miss Sarah Is Thankful Just to Be Here." *The Seattle Times,* November 25, 1999, A1 and A23.

CHAPTER 2

1. Weiss, Rick. "Study: 98,000 Deaths Each Year Are Linked to Medical Mistakes." The *Seattle Times,* November 30, 1999, A1.

2. Northrup, Christiane. *Women's Bodies, Women's Wisdom: Creating Physical and Emotional Health and Healing.* New York: Bantam Books, 1998, 658.

3. Ibid., 168.

4. Goldberg, Burton. *Alternative Medicine Guide to Women's Health.* Tiburon, CA: Future Medicine Publishing, 1998, 102.

5. Catherine Schairer, Ph.D.; Jay Lubin, Ph.D.; Rebecca Troisi, Sc.D.; Susan Sturgeon, Dr.P.H.; Louise Brinton, Ph.D.; Robert Hoover, M.D. "Menopausal Estrogen and Estrogen-Progestin Replacement Therapy and Breast Cancer Risk." *Journal of the American Medical Association,* vol. 283, no. 4, January 26, 2000, 485–491.

6. Haney, Daniel. "Second Heart Study Discounts Estrogen." The *Seattle Times.* March 14, 2000, 1.

7. Ibid., 1.

8. Ibid., 1.

CHAPTER 3

1. Hahnemann, Samuel. *Organon of the Medical Art,* edited by Wenda Brewster O'Reilly. Redmond, WA: Birdcage Books, 1996, 78.

2. Bellavite, Paolo, and Andrea Signorini. *Homeopathy: A Frontier in Medical Science.* Berkeley, CA: North Atlantic, 1995, 68–78.

3. A meta-analysis published in 1997 in the highly respected British medical journal the *Lancet,* which reviewed over one hundred randomized, placebo-controlled trials and concluded that its clinical effects were not due only to placebo (Linde, Klaus, et al. "Are the Clinical Effects of Homeopathy Placebo Effects? A Meta-Analysis of Placebo-Controlled Trials." *Lancet,* vol. 350 [1997]: 834–843).

A review of over one hundred clinical trials in homeopathy conducted between 1966 and 1990, published in the *British Medical Journal* in 1991, which found positive results in 76 percent of the studies for such conditions as flu, hay fever, rheumatoid arthritis, digestive problems, fibromyalgia, infections, psychological problems, and recovery from surgery. (Kleijnen, Paul, Paul Knipschild, and Gerben ter Riet. "Clinical Trials of Homeopathy." *British Medical Journal,* vol. 302 [February 9, 1991]: 316).

The widely publicized study by the renowned French physician and immunologist Jacques Benveniste, published in the prestigious journal *Nature* and replicated at four universities, which proved that the immunoglobulin antibody (IgE) continued to react when exposed to an antigen even after repeated dilutions in water. (Davenas, E., F. Beauvais, J. Amara, M. Robinson, A. Miadonna, A. Tedeschi, B. Pomeranz, P. Fortner, P. Belon, J. Sainte-Laudy, B. Poitevin, J. Benveniste. "Human Basophil Degranulation Triggered by Very Dilute Antiserum Against IgE." *Nature,* vol. 333 [30 June 1988]: 816–818). A subsequent study replicated the data. (Benveniste, J., E. Davenas, B. Ducot, B. Cornillet, B. Poitevin, and A. Spira. "L'agitation de solutions hautement diluees ninduit pas dactivite biologique specifique." *C. R. Academy Science, Paris,* vol. 312, no. 461 [1991]).

Three studies, including a meta-analysis, conducted at the Glasgow Homeopathic Hospital, published in the *Lancet,* found a significantly favorable result in the treatment of 28 patients with hay fever. (Reilly, D., N. G. Taylor, J. H. Beattie, et al. "Is Evidence for Homeopathy Reproducible?" *Lancet,* vol. 344 [1994]: 1601–1606).

4. Ullman, Dana. *The Consumer's Guide to Homeopathic Medicine.* New York: Tarcher/ Putnam, 1995, 36–37.

5. Ibid., 36–37.

CHAPTER 13

1. Northrup, Christiane. *Women's Bodies, Women's Wisdom.* New York: Bantam Books, 1998, 354.

2. Hudson, Tori, N.D. *Women's Encyclopedia of Natural Medicine.* Lincolnwood, IL: Keats, 1999.

3. Northrup, Christiane. *Women's Bodies, Women's Wisdom.* New York: Bantam Books, 1998, 268.

4. Hudson, Tori, N.D. *Women's Encyclopedia of Natural Medicine.* Lincolnwood, IL: Keats, 1999, 143.

5. Northrup, Christiane. *Women's Bodies, Women's Wisdom.* New York: Bantam Books, 1998, 130–131.

6. Hudson, Tori. *Women's Encyclopedia of Natural Medicine.* Lincolnwood, IL: Keats, 1999, 265.

CHAPTER 15

1. Halberstam, Yitta, and Judith Levanthal. *Small Miracles of Love and Friendship: Remarkable Coincidences of Warmth and Devotion.* Holbrook, Mass.: Adams Media Corporation, 1999, 98–101.

CHAPTER 16

1. Godden, Jean. "Random Act Starts Chain of Kindness." The *Seattle Times,* January 7, 2000, B4.

Glossary

aggravation—a temporary worsening of already existing symptoms after taking a homeopathic medicine

allopathic medicine—a type of medical system that uses a different, rather than a similar, medicine to heal

alternative medicine—natural approaches to healing that are nontoxic and safe, including homeopathy, naturopathic medicine, chiropractic, acupuncture, botanical medicine, and many other methods of healing

antidote—a substance or influence that interferes with homeopathic treatment

casetaking—the process of the in-depth homeopathic interview

chief complaint—the main problem that causes a patient to visit a health-care practitioner

classical homeopathy—a method of homeopathic prescribing in which only one medicine is given at a time, based on the totality of the patient's symptoms elicited in an in-depth interview

combination medicine—a mixture containing more than one homeopathic medicine

constitutional treatment—homeopathic treatment based on the whole person, involving an extensive interview and careful follow-up

conventional medicine—mainstream, orthodox, Western medicine

defense mechanism—the aspect of the vital force that maintains health and prevents disease

high-potency medicines—homeopathic medicines of a 200C or higher potency

holistic—a type of medicine, usually practiced by nutritionally oriented medical and osteopathic physicians, that addresses the whole person

homeopathic medicine—a medicine that acts according to the principles of homeopathy

homeopathic practitioner—a practitioner who treats people with homeopathic medicines according to the principles of homeopathic medicine as developed by Samuel Hahnemann

homeopathy—a medical science and art that treats the whole person, based on the principle of like cures like

law of similars—the principle of like cures like

low potency medicines—homeopathic medicines of a 30C or lower potency

materia medica—a book that includes individual homeopathic medications and their indications

minimum dose—the least quantity of a medicine that produces a change in a person who is ill

modality—those factors that make a particular symptom better or worse

naturopathic physician—a physician who has graduated from a four-year naturopathic medical school and who treats the whole person based on the principle of the healing power of nature

nosode—a homeopathic medicine made from the products of disease

os—opening of the cervix

potency—the strength of a homeopathic medicine as determined by the number of serial dilutions and succussions

potentization—the preparation of a homeopathic medicine through the process of serial dilution and succussion

prover—a person who takes a specific homeopathic substance as part of a specially designed homeopathic experiment to test the action of the medicine

provings—the process of testing out homeopathic substances in a prescribed way in order to understand their potential curative action on patients

relapse—the return of symptoms when a homeopathic medicine is no longer acting

repertory—a book that lists symptoms and the medicines known to produce such symptoms in healthy provers or in clinical practice

return of old symptoms—the re-experiencing of symptoms from the past, after taking a homeopathic medicine, as part of the healing process

simillimum—the one homeopathic medicine that most clearly matches the symptoms of the patient and that produces the greatest benefit

single medicine—one single homeopathic medicine given at a time

state—an individual's stance in life; how she approaches the world

succussion—the systematic and repeated shaking of a homeopathic medicine after each serial dilution

symptom picture—a constellation of all of the mental, emotional, and physical symptoms that an individual patient experiences

totality—a comprehensive picture of the whole person: physical, mental, and emotional

vital force—the invisible energy present in all living things that creates harmony, balance, and health

Index

A

Acne rosacea, 183–185
Acne vulgaris, 185–187
Aconite
  fear of flying, 89
  fright, 94
  insomnia, 112
  labor and delivery, 122
  miscarriage, 137
  uses, guidance, 275–276
Aesculus, 102, 276–277
Aggravation, 174
Aloe, 102
Aloe socotrina. See Aloe
Alumina, 117
American arum. *See Caladium*
Animal types, 22
Anorexia. *See* Eating disorders
Antibiotics, 40
Antidoting substances, 175–176
Anxiety, 187–190. *See also* Performance
  anxiety
Apis mellifica
  bee stings, 17–18
  bladder infections, 78
  miscarriage, 137
  uses, guidance, 277–278
Argentum nitricum
  fear of flying, 89
  fright, 94
  performance anxiety, 150

Arnica
  fright, 94
  jet lag, 117
  surgery, 163
  uses, guidance, 278–279
Arsenic. *See Arsenicum album*
Arsenicum album
  fear of flying, 89
  fright, 94
  insomnia, 112
  uses, guidance, 279–280
Aurum metallicum, 98

B

Belladonna
  beastfeeding problems, 84
  mastitis, 127
  menstrual pain, 132
  uses, guidance, 280–281
Bellis perennis, 281–282
Better-sweet. *See Dulcamara*
Birth control. *See* Contraceptives
Bitter cucumber. *See Colocynthis*
Black cohosh. *See Cimicifuga*
Bladder infections, 190–193
Bloodroot. *See Sanguinaria*
Blue cohosh. *See Caulophyllum*
Borax, 89
Breast cancer, 193–196

Breastfeeding problems, 80–85.
See also Mastitis
Breathing, importance, 333–334
Bryonia
beastfeeding problems, 84
mastitis, 127
uses, guidance, 282–283
Bulimia. See Eating disorders
Bushmaster snake. See Lachesis
Business, unfinished, 332

C

Cactus grandifolia, 132, 283–284
Caladium, 167, 284–285
Calcarea carbonica, 84, 90,
285–286
Calcium carbonate.
See Calcarea carbonica
Calcium sulfide. See Hepar sulphuris
Calendula, 163
Candida, 28–29
Cantharis, 78, 286–287
Carnegie, Andrew, 19
Case taking
description, 51–54
icons, 71–72
recording, 56–57
sample, 55–56
symptoms, 53–54
Castor equi, 127, 287–288
Caulophyllum
labor and delivery, 122
miscarriage, 137
uses, guidance, 288–289
Cervical dysplasia.
See Genital warts
Chamomilla
insomnia, 112
menstrual pain, 132
uses, guidance, 289–290
Chamomille. See Chamomilla
Chemotherapy, 40

China
labor and delivery, 122
miscarriage, 137
uses, guidance, 290–291
Chinese medicine, 24
Chiropractic medicine, 24
Cimicifuga
hot flashes, 107
labor and delivery, 122
postpartum depression, 159
uses, guidance, 291–292
Club moss. See Lycopodium
Coal oil. See Petroleum
Cocculus
jet lag, 117
morning sickness, 142
motion sickness, 147
uses, guidance, 292–293
Coffea, 112, 293–294
Colchicum, 142, 295
Collinsonia, 102, 296
Colocynthis, 132, 297
Compassion, 332
Conium, 298
Connectedness, 7
Contraceptives, 40
Conventional medicine
associated deaths, 9
drugs, 10–16
high-tech advances, 9–10
-homeopathy
combining, 36–37
comparison, 38–39
compatible treatments, 40
incompatible treatments, 40
support for, 41
surgery
after effects, 10
over uses, uses, guidance, 12–13
recommendations, 13–14
Corticosteroids, 40
Creativity, enhanced, 6–7
Creator, connecting with, 334–335

Creosote. *See Kreosotum*
Cuttlefish ink. *See Sepia*
Cypripedium, 159

D

Daisy. *See Bellis perennis*
Deadly nightshade. *See Belladonna*
Depression, 196–201
     postpartum, 156–159, 254–256
Diet, healthful, 333
Dilutions, 23–24
Dog's milk. *See Lac caninum*
Drugs. *See* Pharmaceutical drugs
Dulcamara, 84

E

Eating disorders, 201–204
Eczema, 38–39
Emotions
     balance, 6, 28–29
     physical symptoms, 3–4
     subconscious, 32
Endometriosis, 204–206
Energy, 6
Engorgement. *See* Breastfeeding problems
Estrone/follicular hormone. *See Folliculinum*
Exercise, 333

F

Families, relationships, 332
Fear of flying, 86–90
Fibrocystic breasts, 206–208
Fibroids. *See* Uterine fibroids
First-aid, 44
Flexner Report, 19
Flint. *See Silica*
Folliculinum, 154, 299
Food and Drug Administration, 23
Forgiveness, 332
Fright, 91–93

G

Gallstones, 208–210
Gelsemium
     fear of flying, 90
     insomnia, 113
     labor and delivery, 123
     performance anxiety, 150
     uses, guidance, 300–301
Genital warts, 210–212
Gold. *See Aurum metallicum*
Grief, 95–98

H

Hahnemann, Dr. Samuel,
     18–19, 25
Hamamelis, 102, 301–302
Headaches, 212–214
Healing
     chain reaction, 338
     meaning, 336–337
     standards, 6–8
Health, maintaining, 332–333
Heart and Estrogen-Progestin
     Replacement Study, 14
Heart disease, 14–15
Heavy periods.
     See Menstrual problems
Help, asking for, 333
Hemlock. *See Conium*
Hemorrhoids, 99–103
Hepar sulphuris, 127
Herbal medicine, 24
Herpes, 215–217
Herrington, Dr. David, 14
Hippocrates, 18
Holistic medicine, 24
Homeopathy
     acceptance, 26
     as alternative, 34
     approaches, 38–39
     assessing, 34–35

Homeopathy, *continued*
  case taking
    description, 51–54
    recording, 56–57
    sample, 55–56
    symptoms, 53–54
  choosing, 37–38
  chronic conditions, 45–46
  classification, 22–23
  common questions, 177–180
  complements, 331–335
  condition response, 29–30
  -conventional medicine
    combining, 36–37
    comparison, 38–39
    compatible treatments, 39
    incompatible treatments, 40
    support for, 41–42
  cost, 33–34
  curative aspects, 33
  definition, 17–18
  as energy form, 337–338
  essence, 19–20
  first-aid, 44
  guidelines, 46–47
  healing standards, 6–8
  history, 18–19
  holistic aspects, 28–32
  individual aspects, 20, 31
  interview process, 32, 171–173
  mechanisms, 25
  medicines
    administering, 61
    care of, 69
    changing, 65–66
    choosing, 58–60, 73
    cost, 67
    prescription, 173–174
    reactions, 174
    repeating, 64–65
    researching, 72
    self-care kits, 67–69
    symptom effects
      complete relief, 62–63
      no change, 62
      partial improvement, 62
      variable, 63–64
      worsening, 63
  minor illnesses, 44
  natural healing *vs.*, 24
  as ongoing process, 33
  personal story, 45
  practitioners
    primary care, 38
    selecting, 27
    types, 26–27
  preparation, 23–24
  protective effects, 34
  reactions, 175–176
  safety, 30
  second opinions, 175
  severe illnesses, 44–45
  and subconscious, 32–33
  success rate, 177
  typical course, 174–175
  variety, 21–22
Honeybee. *See Apis mellifica*
Hops. *See Bryonia*
Hormone-replacement therapy, 14–16,
    229–230
Hot flashes, 104–108
HRT. *See* Hormone-replacement therapy
Human papilloma virus. *See* Genital warts
Humor, 333
Hydrocortisone, 39
Hypericum, 163
Hysterectomies, 12

I

Icons, description, 70–73
Ignatia
  grief, 98
  insomnia, 113
  miscarriage, 138
  uses, guidance, 302

Incontinence, 217–219
Indian cockle. *See Cocculus*
Infertility, 219–220
Insomnia, 109–113
Interviews, 32
Intimacy, giving to, 334
Ipecac, 142
Irregular periods. *See* Menstrual problems

J

Jet lag, 114–117
Journal of the American Medical
    Association, 14

K

Kahaloa, Sarah, 7–8
Kegel's exercises, 218
King, Martin Luther Jr., 337
Kreosotum
    morning sickness, 142
    PMS, 154
    uses, guidance, 303–304
    vaginitis, 167

L

Labor and delivery, 118–123. *See also*
    Pregnancy-related problems
Lac caninum, 84, 304–305
Lac defloratum, 85
Lachesis
    hot flashes, 107
    PMS, 154
    uses, guidance, 305–306
Lactuca virosa, 85, 305–306
Lady's slipper. *See Cypripedium*
La Leche League, 83
Lark, Susan, 182
Law of Similars, 17–18
Leopard's bane. *See Arnica*
Lifestyles, balanced, 331–335

Lilium tigrinum, 154, 307–308
Love, 331, 335
Lycopodium, 150, 308–309

M

Magnesia phosphoricum, 133, 309–310
Magnesium phosphate. *See Magnesia*
    phosphoricum
Marigold. *See Calendula*
Mastitis, 124–128. *See also* Breastfeeding
    problems
Materia medica, 21
Meadow saffron. *See Colchicum*
Menopause, uses, guidance, 223–231
Menstrual problems, 129–133, 231–234
Mental stability, 6, 32
Mercuric chloride. *See Mercurius*
    corrosivus
Mercurius corrosivus, 78, 310–311
Mineral types, 23
Miscarriages, 134–138, 235–238
Modalities, 53–54
Monkshood. *See Aconite*
Mood swings, 238–240
Morning sickness, 139–143, 240–243
Motion sickness, 144–147

N

Narcotic drugs, 40
Natrum muriaticum, 98, 311–312
Nature, appreciating, 334
Naturopathic medicine
    acne rosacea, 185
    acne vulgaris, 187
    bladder infections, 76–77, 192–193
    breast cancer, 195–196
    breastfeeding problems, 82–83
    depression, 200–201
    description, 24
    eating disorders, 203–204
    endometriosis, 206

Naturopathic medicine, *continued*
  fear of flying, 88
  fibrocystic breasts, 208
  fright, 93
  gallstones, 209–210
  genital warts, 212
  grief, 96–97
  headaches, 214
  hemorrhoids, 101
  herpes, 216–217
  hot flashes, 106
  incontinence, 218–219
  infertility, 220
  insomnia, 111
  jet lag, 115–117
  labor and delivery, 120–121
  low sexual energy, 222
  mastitis, 126
  menopause, uses, guidance, 230–231
  menstrual problems, 131, 234–235
  miscarriages, 136, 237–238
  mood swings, 240
  morning sickness, 141, 242–243
  motion sickness, 146
  osteoporosis, 245
  ovarian cysts, 248
  pelvic pain, 251
  performance anxiety, 149
  PMS, 254
  polycystic ovaries, 248
  postpartum depression, 157–158,
    255–256
  pregnancy, 258
  premenstrual syndrome, 153
  sexual abuses, uses, guidance,
    258–261
  surgery, 162
  uterine fibroids, 264
  vaginismus, 271
  vaginitis, 166, 269
Night-blooming cereus. *See Cactus
    grandifolia*
Northrup, Dr. Christiane, 218

Nux vomica
  hemorrhoids, 103
  insomnia, 113
  menstrual pain, 133
  use, guidance, 312–313

O
Ohio buckeye. *See Aesculus*
Organon of Medicine, 19
Osteoporosis, 243–245
Ovarian cysts, 246–248

P
Patience, 334
Peace of mind, 334
Pelvic pain, 248–251
People, positive, 331
Performance anxiety, 148–150
Peruvian bark. *See China*
Petroleum
  jet lag, 117
  motion sickness, 147
  uses, guidance, 313–314
Pharmaceutical drugs
  advantages, 10–11
  disadvantages, 11–12
  HRT, 14–16
Phellandrium, 128, 314–315
Phosphoric acid, 98
Phosphorus, 163, 315–316
Physical symptoms
  aspects, 3–5
  emotions, 32
  improvement, 6
Phytolacca, 128, 316–317
Plant types, 22–23
Playfulness, 333
PMS. *See* Premenstrual syndrome
Poison nut. *See Nux vomica*
Pokeroot. *See Phytolacca*
Polycystic ovaries, 246–248

Postpartum depression. *See* Depression
The Power of Now, 331
Practitioners
   primary care, 40–41
   selecting, 27
   types, 26–27
Pregnancy-related problems. *See also*
   Labor and delivery
   depression after, 156–159
   morning sickness, 242–243
   treatments, 256–258
Premenstrual syndrome, 151–155,
   251–253
Prescriptions, 173–174
Present, being, 331
Proving, 174
Pulsatilla
   breastfeeding problems, 85
   hot flashes, 107
   labor and delivery, 123
   miscarriage, 138
   PMS, 155
   postpartum depression, 159
   uses, guidance, 317–318
   vaginitis, 167
Purpose, sense of, 7

Q
Quaker's button. *See Nux vomica*

R
Reactions, 174–176
Reeve, Christopher, 336
Relationships, healing, 332
Responsibility, taking, 334
Rudimentary thumbnail of the horse.
   See Castor equi

S
Sabina, 138, 318–319
Safety, 30

Sanguinaria, 107, 319–320
Sanicula, 167
Sarsaparilla, 79, 320–321
Savine. *See Sabina*
Self-care kits, 67–69
Self-treatment
   case taking
      description, 51–54
      recording, 56–57
      sample, 55
      symptoms, 53–54
   chronic conditions, 45–46
   first-aid, 44
   guidelines, 46–47
   minor illnesses, 44
   personal story, 45
   severe illnesses, 44–45
Sepia
   characterization, 21–22
   hot flashes, 108
   labor and delivery, 123
   miscarriage, 138
   morning sickness, 143
   motion sickness, 147
   PMS, 155
   postpartum depression, 159
   uses, guidance, 321–322
   vaginitis, 167
Service, importance, 331–332
Sexual abuses, uses, guidance,
   258–261
Sexual energy, low, 221–222
Silica
   breastfeeding problems, 85
   mastitis, 128
   performance anxiety, 150
   uses, guidance, 323
Silver nitrate. *See Argentum nitricum*
Skimmed milk. *See Lac defloratum*
Small Miracles of Love and
   Friendship, 332
Sodium biborate. *See Borax*
Sodium chloride. *See Natrum muriaticum*

Spanish fly. *See Cantharis*
Spiritual satisfaction, 7
Spiritual separation, 4–5
Spring water. *See Sanicula*
St. Ignatius bean. *See Ignatia*
St. John's wort. *See Hypericum*
Staphysagria, 163
Staphysagria guidance, 324
State, description, 54
Stavesacre. *See Staphysagria*
Stinging nettle. *See Urtica urens*
Stone-root. *See Collinsonia*
Stramonium, 94
Strontium carbonicum, 163
Subconscious, 32–33
Sulphur
  hemorrhoids, 103
  hot flashes, 108
  uses, guidance, 325
Supplements, 333
Suppression, 39–40
Surgery
  after effects, 10
  over uses, uses, guidance, 12–13
  recommendations, 13–14
  treatment, 160–162
Symptoms. *See also specific conditions*
  changing, 66
  comparing, 72
  icon, 70
  modalities, 53–54
  return, 174
  types, 53

T
Tabacum
  morning sickness, 143

motion sickness, 147
  uses, guidance, 326
Thorn apple. *See Stramonium*
Tiger lily. *See Lilium tigrinum*
Tobacco. *See Tabacum*
Tolle, Ekhardt, 331

U
Ullman, Dr. Bob, 223
Unroasted coffee. *See Coffea*
Urtica urens, 85
Uterine fibroids, 261–264

V
Vaginismus, 270–271
Vaginitis, 164–167, 264–269
Veratrum album, 143, 327
Vital force, 28
Vithoulkas, George, 19

W
W. K. Kellogg Foundation, 9
Water dropwort. *See Phellandrium*
White hellebore. *See Veratrum album*
Wild lettuce. *See Lactuca virosa*
Wild licorice. *See Sarsaparilla*
Windflower. *See Pulsatilla*
Witch hazel. *See Hamamelis*
Women's Health Initiative,
  14–15

Y
Yeast infection. *See Candida*
Yellow jasmine. *See Gelsemium*

About the Author

Judyth Reichenberg-Ullman, N.D., D.H.A.N.P., M.S.W., is a licensed naturopathic physician and board-certified diplomate of the Homeopathic Academy of Naturopathic Physicians. She received a doctorate in naturopathic medicine from Bastyr University in 1983 and a master's in psychiatric social work from the University of Washington in 1976. Dr. Reichenberg-Ullman has extensive experience in conventional mental health settings prior to becoming a naturopathic physician.

Past president of the International Foundation for Homeopathy and past faculty member of Bastyr University, she, along with her husband, colleague, and companion Robert Ullman, teaches, writes, and lectures widely. Dr. Reichenberg-Ullman is a frequent guest on radio shows across the United States and was interviewed on National Public Radio's *Talk of the Nation* and *Weekday,* as well as the *Voice of America.* Her articles have been featured in national health magazines such as *Mothering, Natural Health,* and *Let's Live,* and she has been a columnist for the *Townsend Letter for Doctors and Patients* since 1990, as well as for other homeopathic journals.

Dr. Reichenberg-Ullman is coauthor of *Prozac-Free: Homeopathic Medicine for Depression, Anxiety, and Other Mental and Emotional Problems; Ritalin-Free Kids: Safe and Effective Homeopathic Medicine for ADD and Other Behavioral and Learning Problems; Homeopathic Self-Care: The Quick and Easy Guide for the Whole Family;* and *The Patient's Guide to Homeopathic Medicine,* which is used widely by homeopathic practitioners. You can order her books through Picnic Point Press, 131 3rd Avenue, N, Edmonds, WA 98020 at (800) 398-1151, if they are not on the shelf of your local bookstore.

Dr. Reichenberg-Ullman practices at the Northwest Center for Homeopathic Medicine in Edmonds, Washington, and at a satellite clinic in Langley, Washington, and specializes in homeopathic family medicine. She treats patients by telephone consultation when there is no qualified practitioner nearby. For consultations, call (425) 774-5599. Her Web site is www.healthy.net/jrru.

Dr. Reichenberg-Ullman has been married for fourteen years and lives with her husband, their two lovable golden retrievers, and a cat named Creamsicle on Whidbey Island near Seattle, Washington.

ORDER FORM

The Homeopathic Self-Care
Home Medicine Kit

I have designed a compact yellow plastic kit containing the fifty most commonly prescribed homeopathic medicines recommended in this book, all in the 30C potency. The kit measures 5 1/2" long, 3" wide, and 1 3/4" high and is shrink-wrapped. It weighs one pound, and is ideal for traveling.

Please send:

_____ Women's Homeopathic Self-Care Medicine Kit(s).

Name _____

Address _____

City/State/Zip _____

Telephone _____

Visa/MC _____ Exp._____

Signature _____ Check enclosed _____

The price is $85 per kit, with a $5 discount per kit on orders of five or more. Shipping costs $5.00 for the first kit and $2.00 for each additional kit. Washington residents add 8.6% sales tax.

You may also call in or fax your order to:
Whole Woman Homeopathy
131 Third Avenue North, Suite B
Edmonds, WA 98020
phone: 800-398-1151
fax: 425-670-6319

To order through our Web site: www.healthyhomeopathy.com